moon meditations

365 NIGHTTIME REFLECTIONS
FOR A PEACEFUL SLEEP

Jenna R. Calabro

ROCK
POINT
QUARTO.KNOWS.COM
NEW YORK, NY

Dedication

To anyone who has ever looked up at the Moon and felt at home—may you find comfort and beauty in exploring your soul more deeply and connecting with the infinite love of the Universe.

TABLE OF CONTENTS

Introduction

Dear Moon Child,

Do you remember who you are?

Consciously or not, you picked up this book to help you remember.

The external world loves to keep us busy and distracted, constantly pulling us out of alignment with our inner self. This book is here to realign you with your center and spark a deeper connection with your mind, body, and soul. The meditations and images within these pages were created to bring you nightly peace and inspiration along your path of self-discovery and spiritual growth.

It's been a few years now since I started meditating in the traditional sense of the word. But I was just nine years old when I started journaling and have been writing almost every night ever since. It has been a lifelong passion to reflect on my thoughts, feelings, and experiences, seeking to understand myself and this world as profoundly as I possibly can. I have found joy and a deep sense of fulfillment in sharing my reflections in the form of art and words with anyone who resonates or is curious to listen.

My personal experiences, along with studies in music, art, poetry, psychology, mental health counseling, and various forms of spirituality, have all contributed to the creations inside this book. The art and words were made with my own hands, but I can't take all the credit. Really, they are messages from the Universe, and I am just blessed to be the conduit.

This is a 365-day meditation book, each month focusing on a different theme. Each date includes a short phrase accompanied by a few sentences designed to bring you into a space of intimate self-reflection and prepare you for a peaceful sleep. Feel free to use the book as intended (one meditation per evening) or however you please. Follow your intuitive guidance.

WHY MOON MEDITATION?

The art and messages you see here were created between the hours of 10 p.m. and 2 a.m. I believe that nighttime is when the veil between dimensions is thinnest. With the portals between worlds open, we are more curious, receptive, and creative. We think better and we dream bigger.

Meditating during this time, when the Moon is shining, is a reminder of the infinite nature of the Universe and of your conscious place in it. If you allow it, the magic and gentle pull of the Moon's power can guide you into a state of peace, comfort, and openness. Combined with the quiet and stillness that naturally comes at night, you have the perfect recipe for meditation.

The messages in this book are inspired by experiences and self-reflections gathered along my own unique journey. If any of my words do not resonate with you, alter them in whatever way feels comfortable for you. For instance, feel free to substitute "the Universe" with "God," "Source," or whatever else works best for you.

However you choose to use this book, my hope is that the words and images in these pages bring you closer to your most authentic self and to this vast, wild Universe we call home.

Thank you for being here.

Thank you for being you.

With love and gratitude,

Jenna (aka Cecilia Moon)

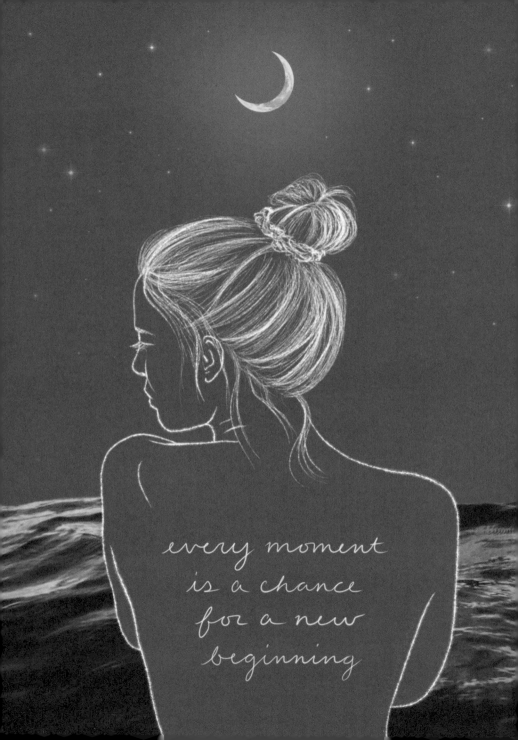

January
EMPOWERMENT

JANUARY 1

Now Is a New Beginning

There is magic right here where you sit. The night overflows with endless possibilities. Every moment carries boundless potential from which you have the power to create change. Now is a new beginning, and you are the creator of that beginning.

✩ .... ✩

JANUARY 2

You Have So Many Gifts

Think of the smallest creatures on the planet—the firefly creating light shows, the spider spinning intricate masterpieces, the caterpillar completely metamorphosizing . . . If even the smallest of creatures has special traits, imagine the gifts that exist within you.

JANUARY 3

There Is Nothing to Prove

You do not owe anyone an explanation of your opinions, your beliefs, or your decisions. No one can decide for you what is right or wrong. Sleep soundly tonight knowing there's nothing to prove to anyone but yourself.

☆ .... ☆

JANUARY 4

You Are a Creator

You were born a creator. Allow yourself to explore whatever you want to create in this life. The more you follow that curiosity, that fire, the closer you will come to know the Universe, and the closer you will come to know your own soul.

JANUARY 5

You Are Infinite Love

The abundance of love that exists in the Universe is beyond comprehension. And because you reflect the Universe, there is no limit to the love that you can nurture within yourself. You carry within you the infinite love of the Universe.

☆ ·· ☆

JANUARY 6

Keep Dreaming

Dreamers are often considered impractical and naïve. But without imagination, there would be no progress in this world. All things begin in the mind before they become tangible. Your dreams are not foolish or futile. Keep dreaming.

JANUARY 7

You Are Limitless

People try to limit you not because of anything to do with you, but because of their own fears. They don't realize they have limited themselves and are projecting their self-limitations onto you. Let them think what they want. You know you are limitless.

☆ .... ☆

JANUARY 8

Determine Your Truth

Not all your thoughts are true. Thoughts only become true when you give them weight and meaning. The more you let your thoughts affect your emotions and behaviors, the more real they will become. Tell yourself tonight, "I have the power to determine my own truth."

JANUARY 9

Everything Is Temporary

The Moon waxes and wanes, moods change, relationships come and go. The ever-evolving nature of life may be scary, but fear doesn't have to be negative. Let it motivate you to make the most of every moment. Use it as fuel to embrace more of what makes you feel alive.

☆ .... ☆

JANUARY 10

Empowerment Is Not Always Loud

Empowerment is keeping peace inside you when there is chaos all around. It is staying true to your own energy rather than matching everyone else's. It is choosing authenticity over acceptance, compassion over judgment, and love over fear.

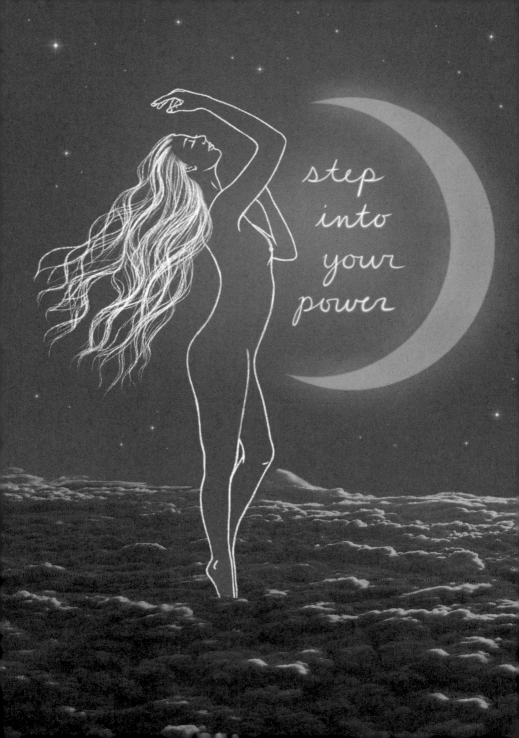

step
into
your
power

JANUARY 11

Step into Your Power

Strip away the noise, the labels, the stories of who you were and who you think you might become. Step into this moment, into the opportunities it holds. Step into your power and embrace the creator you have always been.

☆ .... ☆

JANUARY 12

Freedom Comes from Within

Freedom is a state of mind and a state of being. You get to choose your perspectives, your beliefs, and how you spend your time and energy. Align with your authentic needs and desires and freedom will naturally follow.

JANUARY 13

Express Your Wild

Most of society has lost touch with its true essence. Remember that you are a force of nature, and you have every right to express yourself as such. Before closing your eyes for sleep tonight, imagine yourself as a bird or fairy, and let your wild spirit soar.

☆ .... ☆

JANUARY 14

Invest in Yourself

There is no greater investment than investing in yourself. You are the one and only thing guaranteed to be with you throughout your entire life. Take a chance on yourself. Decorate your mind with beautiful, loving thoughts. Make your inner home a sanctuary of safety and peace.

JANUARY 15

Discover Something New

The vastness of outer space is impossible for the mind to fully comprehend. The oceans, too, are difficult to fathom. There is so much still to explore about the worlds above and below. And what about within you? The soul is vast, too. What inner discoveries can you make tonight?

☆ ....•......... ☆

JANUARY 16

Choose Love

You may not be able to eliminate inner darkness, but you do get to decide how you interact with it. You can choose the energy you want to embody. Acknowledge the shadows but do not feed them with anxious, fearful thoughts. Instead, show them love. Darkness loses its power when the light comes on.

JANUARY 17

Your Truth Is Yours

Close your eyes and picture gentle blue light surrounding your throat. Remind yourself that you have the freedom to choose what parts of yourself you express and with whom. Your truth is yours to protect or to share as you please.

☆ .... ☆

JANUARY 18

Only You Decide

Society sends daily messages that you aren't enough: aren't working hard enough, making enough money, exercising enough, fitting in enough. But you are enough. And only you get to decide the changes you need to make for yourself.

JANUARY 19

You Change the World

It is beautiful to effect change by contributing your knowledge and talents to the world. But your greatest contribution need not be a material one. You affect others through your compassion, authenticity, and everything that makes you who you are. You change the world simply by being yourself.

☆ .... ☆

JANUARY 20

Make Yourself a Priority

You get to decide how much you let others affect your energy. If you feel drained around a particular person, gently move on. Find out what elevates your spirit and do more of that.

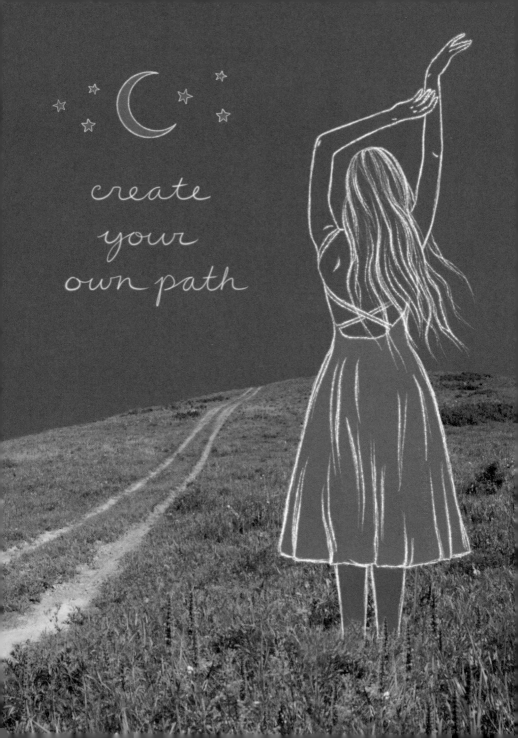

JANUARY 21

Create Your Own Path

You carry inside you a unique signature that cannot be copied. There is no one else with your fingerprints. So why follow in the footsteps of another? You are here for a purpose. Create your own path.

☆ ⋯⋯⋯⋯⋯⋯⋯⋯⋯⋯⋯⋯⋯⋯ ☆

JANUARY 22

Explore

May the fire within you never extinguish. The air may be cold, the earth covered in snow, but there is warmth in your heart. Let your desire to explore the world around you and within you keep you thriving (not just surviving) wherever you may go.

☆ ⋯⋯⋯⋯⋯⋯⋯⋯⋯⋯⋯⋯⋯⋯ ☆

JANUARY 23

Breathe to the Rhythm

As you sit down to meditate tonight, quietly play one of your favorite songs. Choose one that makes you feel inspired yet calm. Follow the beat of the music and breathe in sync with it. Find comfort within its steady rhythm.

JANUARY 24

Remember Where You Came From

You were not always the person you are today. Remember the prior versions of you who struggled with things that now come easily. Go to sleep tonight with compassion for yourself and the journey you have traveled.

☆ ⋯⋯⋯⋯⋯⋯⋯⋯⋯⋯⋯⋯⋯⋯⋯⋯⋯⋯⋯⋯ ☆

JANUARY 25

You Cannot Be Compared

Beauty cannot be defined in only one way. There is equal beauty in assertiveness and reservedness, originality and conventionality, boldness and softness. Your personality is beautiful and cannot be compared.

JANUARY 26

Reality Is Subjective

Everyone lives in a different reality, shaped by their own unique experiences and perception of themselves and the world around them. What makes sense to one person may not to another. Remember that everyone's perception of reality is equally valid.

☆ ⋯⋯⋯⋯⋯⋯⋯⋯⋯⋯⋯⋯⋯⋯⋯⋯⋯⋯⋯⋯ ☆

JANUARY 27

Set Yourself Free

Set yourself free from self-limiting thoughts and beliefs. Free from the noise of others' opinions. Free from past pain and future fear. Free from everything holding you back from blossoming into your highest, most authentic self.

JANUARY 28

You Are Multidimensional

You are a complex being who cannot be labeled or defined. You are the storm and the calm before the storm. You are fire and the water that extinguishes it. You are both light and dark, soft and strong. Let no one make you believe you are too much.

☆ .... ☆

JANUARY 29

You Are Infinite

The journey within teaches you not only about yourself but also about nature, humanity, and the Universe. There is no separation. Everything is one, a part of the great cosmic whole. Your body may be small, but infinity lives within your soul.

JANUARY 30

Imagine the Stars

Have you ever gazed up at the stars and felt humbled by the smallness of your being? Close your eyes and bring that feeling into your meditation. How powerful it is to remember you are a part of such a wild, endless galaxy. And how small your worries will seem in comparison.

☆ ··· ☆

JANUARY 31

Stay Wild, Moon Child

Child of the Universe, never forget that you are a force of nature. You are one with the entire cosmos. Be adventurous. Be curious. Be brave. And never let anyone tame your spirit.

FEBRUARY 1

You Are Enough

There is nothing to prove. When you doubt your beauty, your strength, or your light, look up and remember: you are made of the same stuff as the Moon and stars. You are pure magic, and you are worthy simply by being you.

☆ ·· ☆

FEBRUARY 2

You Are Always Whole

Do you judge the Moon when she is hiding or when she shows only a sliver of her brilliance? No. So why do you judge yourself? Each of your phases is beautiful and important. And you are always whole, even when you don't feel it.

February
SELF-LOVE

FEBRUARY 3

No Feeling Is Permanent

Even in the midst of winter, there is life. Deer roam snow-covered forest floors and fish swim beneath the ice. You may feel cold, restless, or alone, but no feeling is permanent. There is movement happening around you and within you. Find comfort in the ever-changing flow of life.

☆ .... ☆

FEBRUARY 4

You Are Worth the Effort

Many spiders spin a new web every single day. Such work requires patience and discipline, but it is a labor of love. The spider looks after herself to ensure she is properly nourished, and so should you. Take care of yourself. You are always worth the effort.

FEBRUARY 5

Value Yourself

Having dreams is wonderful. But the thrill of reaching milestones is fleeting. The feeling wears off. So just remember, before you start climbing a new mountain, valuing yourself based on external achievements means nothing if you don't first value yourself for who you already are.

✩ ⋯⋯⋯⋯⋯⋯⋯⋯⋯⋯⋯⋯⋯⋯⋯ ✩

FEBRUARY 6

Shine Bright

Never let others' inability to see your light keep you from shining. Your creativity, the uniqueness of your mind, and the empathy in your heart are not dependent on others' acknowledgment or appreciation. You shine bright regardless.

FEBRUARY 7

Prioritize Yourself

It's okay to put your needs first. It's okay to prioritize yourself even when it means disappointing someone else. It's okay to say no and to set boundaries: your energy is precious. It's okay to choose yourself.

☆ ⋯⋯⋯⋯⋯⋯⋯⋯⋯⋯⋯⋯⋯ ☆

FEBRUARY 8

You Are What You Seek

Everything you are looking for already exists within you. The compassion, the peace, the belonging you are seeking can be found right inside your being. Sit with yourself in stillness for a while and you will feel how whole and complete you truly are.

FEBRUARY 9

You Are Art

You are a work of art, created by the Universe with tender love and care. Your strokes, your colors, every part of you was created with intention. You may be ever-evolving but that does not mean you aren't a masterpiece just as you already are.

☆ .... ☆

FEBRUARY 10

Be Kind to Yourself

Are you speaking to yourself kindly and with respect? The thoughts you have about yourself matter. They contribute not only to your self-perception but also to the shaping of your reality. As you fall asleep tonight, make sure your final thoughts are gentle and kind.

FEBRUARY 11

Remember Who You Are

You are so much more than what meets the eye. You are the earth and the sky and everything in between. You carry within you the complexity, beauty, creativity, and unbounded love of the Universe.

☆ ·· ☆

FEBRUARY 12

You Are Your Own Authority

The mind is malleable and easily swayed. Sometimes the opinion of just one person may cause you to question yourself. Keep following your inner guidance and remember that you are the authority of your own life.

FEBRUARY 13

Embrace Your Shadow

The thing about self-love is that it cannot be found by only looking on the surface. You must dig deep into the parts of yourself that have been neglected. Learn to embrace your shadow and you will begin to recognize your light.

☆ .... ☆

FEBRUARY 14

You Have a Purpose

If you feel you do not fit into this world, if your perspectives confuse or disturb others, do not despair. You are not alone, and you are not here in vain. You are being called to share your unique gifts with the world.

FEBRUARY 15

Love Yourself

Loving yourself means letting go. Letting go of the version of you that believes self-love means always putting others first. The version of you that fears being rejected and disliked. The you that feels unworthy of all that you dream of and desire.

☆ .... ☆

FEBRUARY 16

Focus on Yourself

There is nothing selfish about focusing on yourself. The energy you spend on bettering yourself and your life will increase the happiness and peace in your own world and extend into the lives of everyone around you.

FEBRUARY 17

Let Your Thoughts Fall

When unhelpful thoughts enter your mind, gently place your hands in your lap, palms facing up. Now imagine your thoughts falling like snowflakes and settling into your palms. The warmth of your hands melts them, taking away their power and making space for new thoughts to grow.

FEBRUARY 18

Kindness Causes Ripples

Your thoughts and actions matter—not just in your life and the lives of your loved ones, but in the entire world. The kindness you show yourself can cause an entire ripple. Even if you can't see it, everything is connected, like constellations in the night sky.

FEBRUARY 19

Give Yourself Grace

Sometimes your mind will make you feel crazy, broken, or unworthy. But just because you think something doesn't mean it's true. There is no reason to believe every thought you have. Remember that you are human and be compassionate with yourself. You are not meant to be perfect.

☆ .... ☆

FEBRUARY 20

Be There for Yourself

Are you giving yourself the attention and thoughtfulness that you so generously give to others? Be sure not to neglect your own needs. You deserve the same amount of love and care. Nourish your mind and heart.

FEBRUARY 21

Believe in Yourself

Magic is believing in yourself. You were not born with limitations to who you are or what you can create in this life. Limits are learned, and so they can be unlearned. Remember that your potential knows no bounds. You are wildly capable.

✩ ·· ✩

FEBRUARY 22

Appreciate Yourself

Never allow judgment or rejection from others to cloud your own view of yourself. Your vulnerability is beautiful. Be proud of having the courage to express yourself. Appreciate what makes you different and know that every part of you is invaluable.

FEBRUARY 23

You Are Already Perfect

Perfection is an illusion. Think of the Moon, how she appears round and smooth from a distance, but up close has many craters. Do her craters detract from her glow? No, because realness is the true perfection. And through the eyes of the Universe, you are perfect just as you are.

☆ ⋯⋯⋯⋯⋯⋯⋯⋯⋯⋯⋯⋯⋯⋯⋯⋯⋯⋯⋯ ☆

FEBRUARY 24

Give Yourself Love

You are capable of creating the life that you wish for. But you cannot create from a place of lack, desperation, or low self-esteem. You cannot manifest what you feel unworthy of. Give yourself the love you so freely give to others. You are worthy of all your dreams.

FEBRUARY 25

Connect with Your Breath

Sit with yourself tonight in stillness and connect with your breath. Inhale all the things you love about yourself, and exhale your struggles. No matter what you're going through, you can always find comfort and refuge within.

✩ ⋯⋯⋯⋯⋯⋯⋯⋯⋯⋯⋯⋯⋯⋯⋯⋯⋯ ✩

FEBRUARY 26

Connect with Yourself

Loneliness does not necessarily reflect a need for connection with another person. Often what you may desire is love and understanding from yourself. Give yourself what you desire from another, and you will find yourself full once again.

FEBRUARY 27

You Belong Deeply to Yourself

You may feel as though you don't belong in this world. But that is because you are looking for belonging in all the wrong places. There is nowhere out there that is as comforting and as safe as the refuge of your own soul.

☆ ⋯⋯⋯⋯⋯⋯⋯⋯⋯⋯⋯⋯⋯⋯⋯⋯ ☆

FEBRUARY 28

Witness All of You

Let the light in. Let it come in through the cracks, exposing all the dark places. Witness every part of you without ridicule or shame. Everything you see is a natural part of being human. Every aspect of you is deserving of love.

☆ ⋯⋯⋯⋯⋯⋯⋯⋯⋯⋯⋯⋯⋯⋯⋯⋯ ☆

FEBRUARY 29

Welcome Home

You are all that you have been seeking. You are the love, the forgiveness, the peace. You've been so busy looking outside of yourself for the things you need when they've been inside you all along. Let your heart be your home.

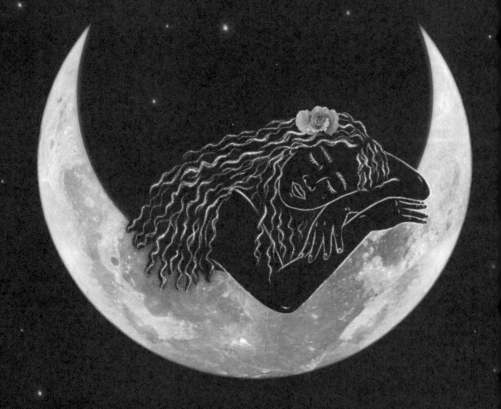

give
yourself
time

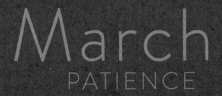

March
PATIENCE

MARCH 1

Give Yourself Time

Your path will unfold in time. It will take time to learn. Time to grow. Time to be present. Time to follow your joy. Time to try and to fall and get up again. Time to rest. Time to forgive and let go.

☆ ·· ☆

MARCH 2

Growth Happens Slowly

Growth does not happen overnight. Be present with the version of yourself that exists today instead of comparing yourself to who you used to be or who you hope to become. You are whole right now in this moment.

MARCH 3

Remember Your Blessings

Where might your impatience come from? Are you afraid that your desires will never arrive? Open your mind and heart. Be curious about what the Universe has in store for you. Remember the blessings you already have, and your grateful energy will attract even more.

MARCH 4

Imagine a Sunset

When you watch a sunset, do you ask the sky to hurry up and change? No, you watch in admiration as the colors transition from blue, to yellow, to orange, pink, and purple. Imagine a sunset tonight and appreciate the pace of your own transformation, too.

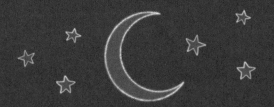

MARCH 5

Simply Allow

Before meditating, open a door or window and feel the night air. Is the temperature warm or cool? Do you notice a breeze touching your skin? And can you observe without forming an opinion? Can you simply allow what is? Carry this perspective with you into your meditations.

MARCH 6

Appreciate the Journey

You may not like your current situation. But sometimes you are where you are because you are being guided to learn what you need to grow. Lean into this present moment and the lessons that it brings.

MARCH 7

Practice Gratitude

Before going to sleep tonight, reflect on everything you were grateful for throughout your day. Remind yourself of the people and things in your life that make you feel blessed and abundant. When there is gratitude in your heart, what you have will always be enough.

☆ .... ☆

MARCH 8

Release Old Ways

Most habits do not change overnight. Your body may need to practice what your mind already knows. Give yourself time to release old ways of being. Be patient as you learn new patterns that will be healthier for your mind, body, and sprit.

MARCH 9

This Moment Is Enough

When impatience knocks at your door, it is a sign that you do not fully trust yourself or the Universe. You are deserving of your desires, and blessings are on their way to you. But until you believe it, this moment will never be enough.

☆ ·· ☆

MARCH 10

The Answer Will Come

If nothing seems to make sense right now, give your mind a break. There may be a lesson in your current situation, but trying too hard to understand only results in inner struggle. Release the desire to control. Know that the answer will come in time.

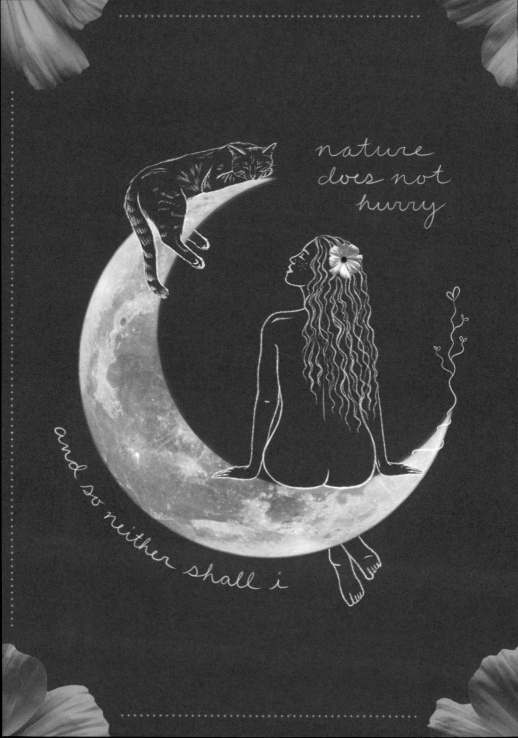

nature
does not
hurry

and so neither shall i

MARCH 11

Nature Does Not Hurry

Nature has so much to teach: Presence. Persistence. Patience. Nature knows that everything happens when it's supposed to. Nature trusts the process. And you are nature, aren't you? So why should you live any differently?

☆ .... ☆

MARCH 12

Be with Yourself Now

Be with yourself in this precious moment. Be with yourself in the space between who you are and who you are becoming. Cherish who you are right here, right now; you will never be this version of you again.

MARCH 13

Meet Yourself Here

Sometimes the experience that crosses your path is not what you want, but rather what you need. Slow down and meet yourself where you are. Reflect on what is troubling you and ask yourself, "What is this trying to teach me?"

☆ ·· ☆

MARCH 14

Nothing Is in Vain

Starting something new often feels like starting from scratch. But nothing you've learned or experienced has been in vain. It has all led you to be the person you are today. And you are kinder, stronger, and wiser for it all.

MARCH 15

Energy Cannot Be Forced

You cannot manifest abundance into your life from a place of impatience or desperation. Energy moves in its own way—it cannot be forced or coerced. Rain will always fall down from the heavens, and flowers bloom up toward the Sun. Lean into the natural movement of life.

☆ .... ☆

MARCH 16

You Are Making Progress

Practice does not make perfect, but it does make progress. Every night you sit down to meditate, you train yourself to be comfortable with slowness, silence, and simplicity. Your thoughts will become quieter, and peace will become louder. Keep going, you are growing.

MARCH 17

Seek Joy in the Ordinary

Humans spend so much time waiting: for happiness, for love, for the next vacation. But big moments pass in the blink of an eye, and you are back to ordinary life. Seek joy in the small things, and your life will be full of magic.

☆ .... ☆

MARCH 18

Slow Down

The mind loves to play tricks. It may try to make you believe that being present is fruitless and unproductive. But action is not the only path toward growth. There is also growth in resting, slowing down, and embracing this moment.

MARCH 19

Be Content

There is always more to be learned, to be bought, to be experienced. Growth in all its forms never ends. But if you are always wanting more, you will never be content with what you already have. Peace is found right here in this moment.

☆ .... ☆

MARCH 20

Believe in Yourself

Impatience implies a lack of trust in your ability to cocreate with the Universe. When you are patient, you believe in yourself and know that everything happens in its own divine time. Trust that you are capable of achieving the life of your dreams.

MARCH 21

Be Patient with Yourself

Just because you can't yet see growth materializing in the physical world doesn't mean you aren't growing. Some plants build an entire root system beneath the earth before they begin to reach up toward the Sun. Allow yourself the time and space to grow at your own pace.

☆ .... ☆

MARCH 22

Be Here Now

Impatience clouds your present and your future. When your focus is on an anticipated outcome, you miss the blessings that are right before your eyes, and you close yourself off to future possibilities. Be grateful for what you have in this moment.

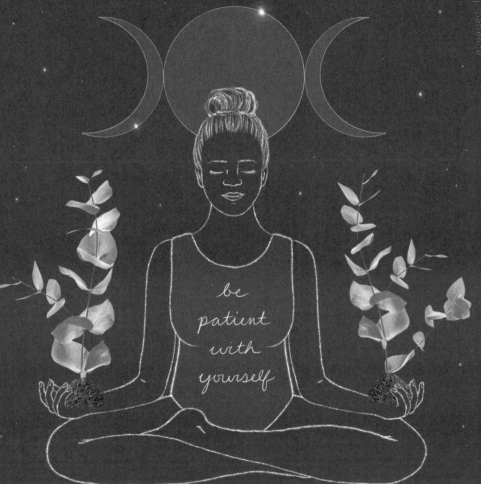

be
patient
with
yourself

MARCH 23

Trust the Process

May the Universe be your blanket tonight. Allow it to protect and comfort you through whatever you are experiencing. Let its gentle weight serve as a reminder for you to slow down. The Universe is always here to support you, and there is no need to hurry when you trust the process.

MARCH 24

You Are Worthy

Are you attaching your worth to a desired outcome? Do you believe that when a certain blessing or milestone arrives, then you will be more valuable or important? The Universe needs no proof of your worthiness. There is no reason to rush.

MARCH 25

Let the Universe Surprise You

You think you want to know how things will turn out, but do you, really? Are you listening to your own authentic voice, or are you listening to fear? Stay curious. Stay open. The Universe may have something in mind for you that is better than you've imagined for yourself.

✩ .... ✩

MARCH 26

Release Your Worries

If you are able, go outside tonight. Let your bare feet touch the earth. Send your worries down through your body and into the ground beneath you. Let Mother Earth do her thing, breaking down your worries so they might decompose and create something new and beautiful.

MARCH 27

Affirm Your Patience

What is something you are struggling to be patient with? Affirm to yourself, "I allow _____ to arrive in its own time." Say this phrase over and over, feeling it become more and more powerful. Repeat until you truly believe the words you are speaking.

☆ .... ☆

MARCH 28

Cultivate Patience

Draw your attention towards the quality of your movements tonight. Position yourself thoughtfully in your seat. Close your eyes gently and breathe slowly. Moving in this way nurtures your body and deepens the bond between yourself and the Universe.

MARCH 29

Heal at Your Own Pace

Your mind may be working through something that your heart is not yet ready to receive. There is no right or wrong way to feel. Give yourself all the time and space you need to heal in whatever way is best for you.

✩ ·· ✩

MARCH 30

Gratitude Is Everything

When you cease thinking about what is yet to come, you become aware of all that you already have. Tune into that awareness. Let it settle on your skin and sink into your bones. There is so much to be grateful for.

✩ ·· ✩

MARCH 31

Let Growth Unfold

There will be times when you feel you are moving backward, unraveling the progress you've made. But just because your life moves linearly from birth to death doesn't mean growth moves the same. Growth unfolds in its own way.

APRIL 1

Share Your Authentic Self

There are endless stars in the sky, yet no two are exactly alike. The Universe doesn't replicate; it creates what is needed. Each star plays an important role, just as you bring to the world something original and special just by being you.

✩ ······································· ✩

APRIL 2

Love Yourself

You bring so much goodness to this world, simply by being your magnificent self. You are beautiful and brave for striving to grow every day, and for learning to love yourself every step of the way.

April
AUTHENTICITY

APRIL 3

Return Inward

Explore, seek knowledge, be curious about others' views and ideas. But always return inward. Be still with yourself and listen to the quiet voice underneath all the noise. Listen and remember that only you can decide who you want to be.

☆ .... ☆

APRIL 4

You Are Not Too Much

You will be too much for some people. They will think you are too loud, too quiet, too harsh, too soft. But you were not created to please others. You were created to be you. Stay true to yourself.

APRIL 5

Celebrate Yourself

Celebrate every accomplishment, big and small. Celebrate especially the ones that no one else sees. Celebrate your courage to express yourself. Celebrate your strength. Celebrate the beautiful energy that you give to the world.

☆ .... ☆

APRIL 6

Focus on You

You are here to understand yourself, not to be understood by others. Instead of focusing on the perception of you through the eyes of another, bring the focus back to yourself. Remember that people can only meet you as deeply as they've met themselves.

APRIL 7

Your Glow Will Return

If you don't feel fully like yourself tonight, that's okay. The Moon does not always feel like herself, either. Sometimes she is eclipsed by the Sun or covered by dark clouds. But she knows that the blanket of gray is not here to stay. She will glow again soon, and so will you.

☆ ·· ☆

APRIL 8

Do Not Fear Rejection

When you allow the fear of rejection to hold you back, you unconsciously choose rejection: you reject yourself. Embrace what makes you, you. Some people may not like you, and that's okay. Let them go and those who are meant to be in your life will find you.

APRIL 9

Never Apologize for Being Yourself

There is no such thing as shining too brightly. You have so much to offer this world, and it is not your responsibility to dim yourself to make others more comfortable. There is no guilt or shame in being who you are.

☆ .... ☆

APRIL 10

You Do Not Need Permission

The truth is there will always be people who do not see, appreciate, or value you. Do not allow fear of rejection to water down your authenticity. Rain does not apologize for the way it flows, nor does thunder apologize for its roar. You do not need permission to be yourself.

APRIL 11

Choose Yourself

Take a moment to give yourself a hug. Remind yourself that you are safe in your body, mind, and heart. It can be challenging to shed the layers you've built to protect yourself but, the more you do so, the more you will uncover who you truly are inside. Keep choosing yourself.

☆ .... ☆

APRIL 12

You Are So Brave

Society is constantly trying to turn you into something you are not: to change the way you look, the food you eat, your perspectives, and your values. It is not easy to sacrifice acceptance and understanding for authenticity. You are so brave for being who you are.

APRIL 13

Own Your Authority

When you express yourself honestly, your inner critic may show up. But that doesn't mean you have to listen. The less power you give your inner critic, the less power it will have over you. You own the authority over your own life.

☆ .... ☆

APRIL 14

Your Authenticity Helps Others

Be fearless in embodying your truest expression, even when it means being misunderstood or rejected. Your authenticity not only heals you but also paves the way for others to see their own unique light. Your authentic self is your greatest gift to the world.

APRIL 15

Embrace Your Uniqueness

Embrace what makes you different. Embrace your quirks, your contradictions, and your multidimensionality. The more you understand and love yourself, the less it will matter to you whether others see and understand you.

☆ ·· ☆

APRIL 16

You Have the Power

You are free to be you in whatever way you choose. You have the power to say yes, to say no, to connect deeply, or to create a boundary. You can be brave and expressive or brave and private. The choice is yours.

APRIL 17

You Are a Constellation

Envision yourself as a constellation, a collection of stars in the sky. There are aspects of you that you've carried since birth, others that are malleable and ever-changing, and still more that are yet to be explored. Be curious about all that makes you, you.

☆ .... ☆

APRIL 18

Stay True to Yourself

There is no shame in holding back your authentic truth when you do not feel safe to share. The degree to which you share yourself with others has no bearing on your level of authenticity. You have a right to your privacy. All that matters is you are true to yourself.

APRIL 19

Learn from the Wolf

Wolves are misunderstood creatures—not cruel and dangerous, but loyal, nurturing, and fearful of humans. Yet wolves do not wonder what humans think of them. (Even if they could, why should they?) Like a wolf, be unbothered by the opinions of others. Keep on living your truth.

☆ .... ☆

APRIL 20

Show Up

Do not trade your authenticity for approval. You were not created to fit in. You were created to be you, and authenticity is never worth sacrificing. Show up for yourself, and for those who need your gifts.

APRIL 21

Align with Your Higher Self

Anytime you feel lost, be still and go within. Nurture any parts of you that you may have left behind. Know that your most authentic, divine self is always there, ready to embrace you at any moment. You are never alone.

☆ ·· ☆

APRIL 22

You Know You Best

Always remember that you are the one who knows you best. Listen to the wisdom of those whose help you seek out, but always come back to yourself. Only you hold the energy to transform into the most authentic and empowered version of yourself.

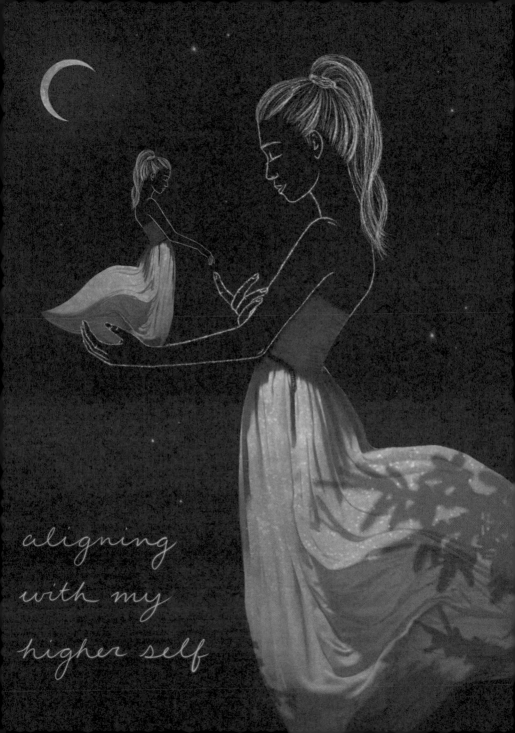

aligning

with my

higher self

APRIL 23

Vulnerability Is Beautiful

Vulnerability gently forces you to face discomfort and fear, opening a path for growth and deeper levels of trust. It allows for genuine connection, making way for love to blossom between yourself, others, and the Universe.

☆ .... ☆

APRIL 24

See Yourself Clearly

As you meditate tonight, picture yourself through the eyes of a loved one. Remember any words they've shared that lovingly suggest where you might benefit from growth. Consider applying this information to your current situation, to help you see more clearly.

APRIL 25

You Are Free to Change

You do not need permission to change. Just as your body is in a continual state of growth and renewal, so are your mind and soul. Recreate yourself as many times as you need. The only approval you need is your own.

☆ .... ☆

APRIL 26

The Moon Does Not Apologize

The Moon does not apologize for the way she glows. She does not feel shame when she is overshadowed by the Sun, or guilt when she causes the waves to crash loudly against the shore. Like the Moon, allow yourself to fully embody who you are meant to be.

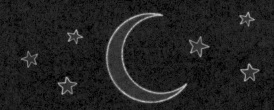

APRIL 27

Enjoy Your Freedom

People may be bothered when they see you moving differently from the crowd. Do not let their discomfort hold you back. Do not let their judgment influence the way you move. You've worked hard to create space for yourself to be authentic and free. Enjoy it.

APRIL 28

Do Not Wait

Do not wait around for others to accept you. Be yourself now. The hurt that may come with being judged or rejected is worth the peace and freedom that come with embodying your most authentic self.

APRIL 29

Your Light Is Needed Here

It is natural to want to be liked and accepted by others. But when conforming to others' views and expectations comes at the expense of your authentic self, you do both yourself and the world a disservice. Give yourself permission to share your light.

☆ ·· ☆

APRIL 30

Come as You Are

Be brave enough to show up in all your realness, your rawness, your vulnerability. Let go of the idea that you are not enough just as you are. You were not made to be perfect; you were made to be you.

MAY 1

You Are Forever Becoming

Growth has no goal or destination. There is no time line or linear path to follow. Allow yourself to travel in your own time and in your own way. There is beauty to be found in the never-ending nature of growth.

☆ ⋯⋯⋯⋯⋯⋯⋯⋯⋯⋯⋯⋯⋯⋯⋯⋯⋯⋯⋯⋯ ☆

MAY 2

Your Journey Is Yours

Your journey is uniquely yours. There is no reason to compare your growth to anyone else's, and no need to worry about how or when you will blossom. Keep reaching for what makes you feel alive, and growth will naturally transpire.

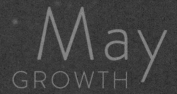

May
GROWTH

MAY 3

Be Curious

When challenging thoughts arise within you, be curious about where they come from. Ask yourself why you believe them to be true. Ask yourself why you've allowed them to shape your perception of yourself and the world around you.

☆ ·· ☆

MAY 4

Flowers Do Not Compete

Flowers do not compete with one another. They are not in a race to see who can grow the fastest or fullest. Just like a flower, navigate your twists and turns without measuring your path against the path of others. There is no reason to compare.

MAY 5

Settle into Space

Have you ever stood in the middle of a desert? No matter in which direction you look, there is an endless expanse of earth and sky. There is little movement, little distraction, nothing obscuring your view. Visualize a desert now. Acclimate yourself with the openness and stillness that surrounds you.

✩ ·· ✩

MAY 6

Unlearn What Doesn't Fit

Growth requires unlearning. Unlearning what was projected onto you from those who didn't know any better. Unlearning the habits and patterns you developed to keep yourself safe. Unlearning what prevents your blossoming. Unlearning so that you can find your way back home.

MAY 7

Lean into Discomfort

There are times for holding on and there are times for letting go. Do not allow fear to dictate which path you take. Often the comfortable option is not for your highest good. Be open to the growth that comes with discomfort. Beauty awaits you on the other side.

☆ .... ☆

MAY 8

Your Beliefs Shape Your Reality

You get to choose the direction of your attention and energy. You decide which perspectives you hold and which ones you throw away. Your beliefs shape your reality, and what you focus on will grow.

MAY 9

Choose to See the Good

Having a positive outlook does not mean ignoring or running away from challenging emotions and experiences. Rather, it means flipping your perspective and choosing to see the good that can be found in every situation.

☆ .... ☆

MAY 10

There Are No Mistakes

Some experiences lead you down a path you do not wish to follow, and it's okay to wish you had chosen otherwise. But realize that all experiences are okay. All roads bring you closer to yourself.

MAY 11

Honor Your Truth

How can you honor your truth? Live in alignment with your values. Express yourself even when you risk being misunderstood or rejected. Respect yourself, your ideas, and your emotions. Set healthy boundaries. Choose authenticity over relatability and trust over fear.

☆ .... ☆

MAY 12

Bloom

Your potential for growth is greatly influenced by where you choose to plant roots and who you allow onto your soil. Plant yourself where you want to bloom, and do not let others block your view of the Sun.

MAY 13

Follow Your Joy

It's wonderful having goals to grow and work toward. But be mindful not to lose touch with your reasons for having goals in the first place. Remember, life is about the journey, not the destination. Make sure the journey brings you joy.

☆ ·· ☆

MAY 14

Spiral into Growth

The natural world is full of spirals, from DNA to nautilus shells to weather patterns to entire galaxies. Movement happens in spirals, growth working inwards, bringing you closer and closer to your soul with every step you take.

MAY 15

Keep Your Balance

Keep your feet on the ground and your eyes on the stars. You cannot grow without roots, but neither can you grow without dreams. Nourish yourself with both and you will continue to bloom.

☆ ··· ☆

MAY 16

You Can't Change Others

People grow at their own pace. You can't change them, and your wish for them to change shows you more about yourself than about them. Accept them for who they are and know you will find others to travel alongside you on your journey of self-discovery.

MAY 17

Be Proud of Your Path

Starting something new can be overwhelming. But you are not starting over. Regardless of the subject at hand, your life experience is relevant. You carry now so much knowledge and wisdom that you didn't have before. Be proud of the path you've traveled.

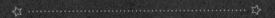

MAY 18

Be Kind

The truth is you never really know what someone is going through. So be kind. Smile at strangers. Look people in the eye. When you see something beautiful about someone, tell them. It may mean more to them than you will ever know.

MAY 19

It's Okay to Rest

Society has created a culture that emphasizes action over reflection. Are you internalizing that belief? Remember that rest is necessary. You are not defined by how many things you do or how often you do them. Sleep soundly tonight knowing it's okay to just be.

☆ ⋯⋯⋯⋯⋯⋯⋯⋯⋯⋯⋯⋯⋯⋯⋯⋯ ☆

MAY 20

Keep Learning

The Universe is your mirror. Every place is a world to explore. Every person is your teacher. Every moment is a chance to look at your reflection and discover more about yourself. Open up your senses and be curious about all there is to learn.

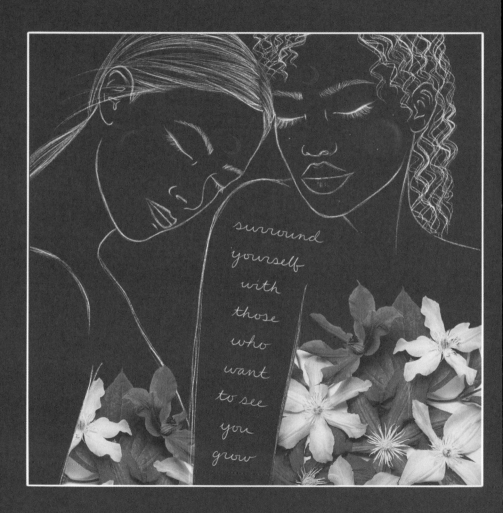

surround
yourself
with
those
who
want
to see
you
grow

MAY 21

Support Each Other's Growth

Surround yourself with those who want to see you grow. Foster connections that inspire authenticity and motivate you to embody the best version of yourself. Invest your time and energy into those who offer the same openness and acceptance that you offer them.

☆ ⋯⋯⋯⋯⋯⋯⋯⋯⋯⋯⋯⋯⋯⋯⋯⋯ ☆

MAY 22

Take a Look Back

The path of growth is long and it's easy to get caught up in all the things you have yet to accomplish. So, when you find yourself lost in worry and self-doubt, pause for a moment. Pause and remember just how far you have come.

☆ ⋯⋯⋯⋯⋯⋯⋯⋯⋯⋯⋯⋯⋯⋯⋯⋯ ☆

MAY 23

Nourish Yourself

Take a nap in the warm sunshine. Relax with a bath. Listen to music. Do whatever it is that fills you up. You cannot grow if you do not take care of yourself.

MAY 24

You Cannot Fail

There is no such thing as failure. Maybe you learned a lesson or maybe you discovered how brave and resilient you are. Find value in everything and your life will be full of meaning.

☆ ⋯⋯⋯⋯⋯⋯⋯⋯⋯⋯⋯⋯⋯⋯⋯⋯⋯ ☆

MAY 25

Aim Higher

Often what feels like rejection isn't truly a loss. Rejection is the Universe's way of guiding you in a different direction. You are wildly capable of achieving your goals, but sometimes you unconsciously limit yourself. You may just need a nudge from the Universe: Aim higher.

MAY 26

Remember Your Ancestors

Reflect on your ancestors tonight. Think of all they endured and accomplished to improve life for themselves and their loved ones. Summon their strength and resilience to help you face your own challenges. They are always there to support you in spirit.

☆ ⋯⋯⋯⋯⋯⋯⋯⋯⋯⋯⋯⋯⋯ ☆

MAY 27

Your Subconscious Is Powerful

What comforting thought do you most need to hear tonight? Whisper it to yourself now. The thoughts you have right before bedtime carry great power. They will be embedded into your subconscious mind, working their magic while you sleep.

MAY 28

Take Care of Yourself

What is deterring you from taking a break? Are you equating your self-worth with your level of productivity? You do not always have to be doing and achieving for growth to occur. Remember that rest is productive, too.

☆ .... ☆

MAY 29

Your Best Is Enough

You do not need to try so hard. Tune into the parts of you that feel stressed, unworthy, or sad. Breathe in the uncomfortable feelings and then release them with your exhale. Remind yourself that your best is more than enough.

MAY 30

There Is No Limit

You are not a problem that needs fixing. You are not a work in progress. You have always been complete and whole. There is no limit to your potential, and you can be content with who you are while still striving to be better.

✧ .... ✧

MAY 31

Small Things Matter

Growth lives in the small things. In the way you speak to yourself, the pause before you react, the way you look at yourself in the mirror. Bring awareness to the little things and watch yourself begin to bloom.

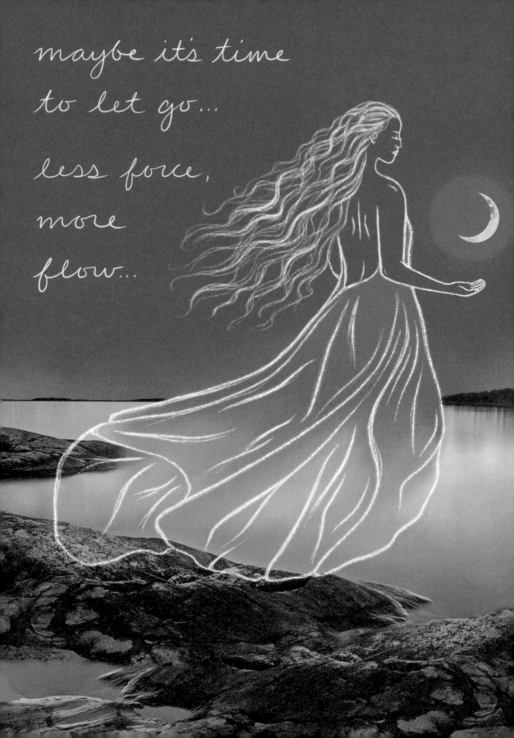

maybe it's time
to let go...

less force,
more
flow...

June
FLOW

JUNE 1

Less Force, More Flow

A boat slowly glides over the water. The boat is empty. There are no motors attached or rowers inside. It does not need to be pushed. Now close your eyes and picture yourself as that boat. Know you are supported. You will get wherever you need to go. Lean back and enjoy the ride.

JUNE 2

You Are Weightless

While you meditate tonight, picture a balloon in your lap. Tune into any unwanted thoughts and imagine sending them down inside the balloon. When you are ready, release the balloon into the air. Without these thoughts, you are liberated, and nothing can hold you down.

✩ ·· ✩

JUNE 3

Let Go

Blessings do not arrive by force or through desperation. They do not come in when you've drained your energy or when you're holding tightly to a desired outcome. Blessings flow when you let go and believe that you are worthy of everything you desire.

JUNE 4

Let Your Spirit Run Free

Imagine yourself as a fish or dolphin, playing in the sea.
Move with the wind and the waves. Let the Sun kiss your
skin. Let the Moon keep you safe. You are wild and free,
and you are only as limited as you believe yourself to be.

☆ ·· ☆

JUNE 5

Let the Energy Flow

Energy is not meant to stay stagnant. It is designed to
keep moving. Allow your emotions to flow through you like
water. Let your thoughts float along the wind. Remember
that everything is temporary. This moment will pass. Let
it all flow.

JUNE 6

Visualize Yourself Sleeping

As you meditate tonight, imagine yourself asleep. See how comfortable and peaceful you look. Notice the steady rhythm of your breath. Bring to bed with you tonight this image you've captured in your mind, and your sleep will be long and peaceful.

✩ ⋯⋯⋯⋯⋯⋯⋯⋯⋯⋯⋯⋯⋯⋯⋯⋯ ✩

JUNE 7

Be Open

It's comforting to see a clear path ahead. To know exactly where you are going and exactly how you will get there. But no matter how much you plan, surprises always come. So, live now, and be open to what the Universe might have in store for you.

JUNE 8

Laugh with the Universe

Invite amusement into your meditation tonight. When you feel out of control, when things don't go according to plan, can you find humor in the situation? You are living on a floating rock in outer space, after all . . . maybe not everything has to be so serious.

JUNE 9

Light Attracts Light

There is no need to chase anything. What you desire will not arrive through force or desperation. Worry and fear will only bring more worry and fear. Embody the energy of that which you desire. Embody kindness, openness, and love. Light attracts light.

JUNE 10

Release Control

There is a natural rhythm to everything that cannot be coerced or controlled. Energy moves in its own way, and you can either fight it and cause yourself needless suffering, or simply go along for the ride. The choice is yours.

JUNE 11

You Can't Miss Your Destiny

What is meant for you will not pass you by. There is no need to chase anything, and no need to force anything. Keep aligning with the best version of yourself, and your best life will naturally find you.

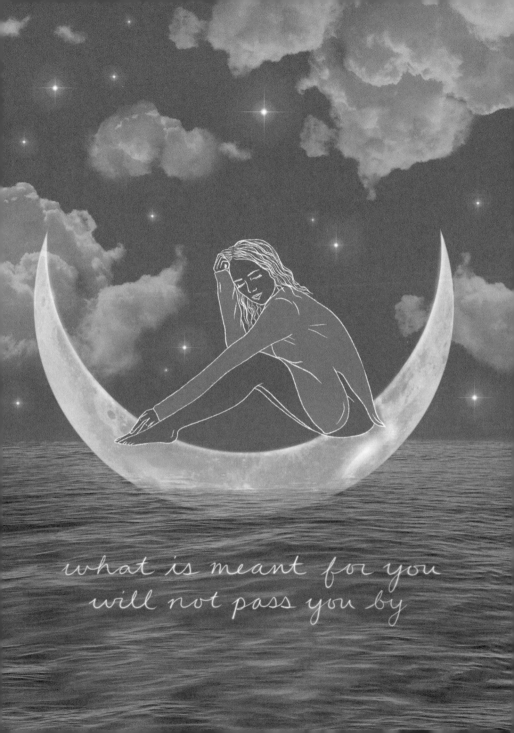

JUNE 12

Notice Movement

When you feel confused or stuck, step outside. Walk around and feel the movement of your feet over the earth. Notice the buzz of insects or birds, the rustle of leaves, the wind in your hair. There is always movement happening, outside you and within you, no matter how stuck you feel.

✩ .... ✩

JUNE 13

Feel the Discomfort

You may feel resistance toward things that are healthy for you. Breaking patterns that have guided your life for a long time is not a comfortable process. But feeling the discomfort is your ticket to the positive change that awaits you on the other side.

JUNE 14

Observe without Forcing

Place your hand over your heart and feel its steady beating. Feel the rise and fall of your chest and stomach as you breathe. Simply observe, without forcing anything. Learn to ride the waves and you will gain courage, strength, and compassion.

☆ ⋯⋯⋯⋯⋯⋯⋯⋯⋯⋯⋯⋯⋯⋯ ☆

JUNE 15

Release Your Thoughts

It may be difficult to quiet your mind. You may think certain thoughts into circles. You may beat yourself up for falling into familiar and unproductive patterns. Know that whatever you are thinking about will resolve in time. Take a breath and release what doesn't serve you.

JUNE 16

Flow with Your Phases

There is a natural rhythm to everything. Think of the tides and the phases of the Moon. Push against the waves and life will keep you stuck. But allow yourself to ride the waves, and you will always move forward.

JUNE 17

Appreciate Everything

Just because you don't like something doesn't mean you can't appreciate it. Just because an emotion or experience is challenging or painful doesn't mean you cannot gain knowledge, strength, and gratitude for the lessons learned.

JUNE 18

Welcome New Energy

Sometimes you hold on to people for longer than you are meant to. But letting go is not selfish, or beneficial for only you. Letting go also honors the other person. It creates space for both of you to bring new, authentic energy into your life.

☆ ⋯⋯⋯⋯⋯⋯⋯⋯⋯⋯⋯⋯⋯⋯⋯⋯ ☆

JUNE 19

Practice Awareness

Observe the sensations within and around you. What do you notice? How do you feel? Awareness brings you closer to this moment, connecting you with yourself and with the Universe. Allow awareness to align you with stillness, truth, and peace.

JUNE 20

Allow Your Humanness

When your thoughts or mood change from moment to moment, know there is nothing wrong with you. You are simply aware of different energies floating around you and flowing through you. Allow yourself to experience the full spectrum of what it means to be human.

✧ ⋯⋯⋯⋯⋯⋯⋯⋯⋯⋯⋯⋯⋯⋯⋯⋯⋯ ✧

JUNE 21

Have Faith in the Tides

Moments of bliss may feel fleeting, while challenging ones may seem to last forever. But all feelings ask to be felt, so lean into this moment, this feeling. Like a wave it will come, and then it will go. Have faith in the ebb and flow.

✧ ⋯⋯⋯⋯⋯⋯⋯⋯⋯⋯⋯⋯⋯⋯⋯⋯⋯ ✧

JUNE 22

Let Go of Expectation

Release your assumptions of how things will turn out. Let go not out of fear of being disappointed or hurt, but out of curiosity, openness, and trust. Let go with a genuine desire to discover what the Universe has in store for you.

have
faith
in the
ebb &
flow

JUNE 23

Do Not Be Defined

Be mindful of creating an identity from your thoughts and feelings. They do not define or control you. Reframe your way of thinking (for instance, you are not an anxious person, you are a person experiencing anxiety). Your thoughts and feelings are giving you a temporary experience to help you learn, heal, and grow.

☆ ⋯⋯⋯⋯⋯⋯⋯⋯⋯⋯⋯⋯⋯⋯⋯⋯⋯⋯ ☆

JUNE 24

Release

Release all that is not yours to carry. Notice any tension in your body, breathe deeply, and you will become aware of what you've been holding on to. Imagine the stuck energy flowing out into the Universe, or down into the earth below you.

JUNE 25

Nothing Is Permanent

Not everyone is meant to be a part of your journey forever. People stay for as long as they serve a purpose in your life, and you in theirs. Do not be saddened when your time together expires. Let impermanence teach you appreciation and gratitude.

☆ .... ☆

JUNE 26

Create Balance

Feelings are fleeting and thoughts can easily change. Do not identify yourself so strongly with a particular idea or perspective that you are unable to see value in another. There is peace and wisdom to be found in remaining open.

JUNE 27

Move with Ease

There are infinite opportunities to choose differently. You can choose to let your thoughts flow through you instead of fixating on them. You can choose to feel your emotions instead of running away. You can choose to move with ease in every moment.

☆ .... ☆

JUNE 28

Inhale Love, Exhale Fear

There is tension in your body waiting to be released. Allow your breath to aid you in letting go. Breathe in what you would like to attract and breathe out what no longer serves you. Inhale trust, exhale doubt. Inhale love, exhale fear.

JUNE 29

Allow Contrast

You can only know something by its opposite. You know light because you know darkness, peace because you know chaos, and love because you know fear. Allow contrast, outside you and within you. Let both exist simultaneously. This is how you flow with the Universe.

✩ ·· ✩

JUNE 30

Open Your Heart

Give yourself permission to leave behind that which no longer serves you. You have to release stale energy to clear space for new, fresh energy to flow in. Open your heart and welcome whatever comes, knowing it is always for your highest good.

JULY 1

You Are Free

In this moment, you are free. Free from past regrets and fears of the future. Free from the judgments and expectations of others. Free from your own self-imposed limitations. Free from everything weighing you down and keeping you from embodying your most magnificent self.

☆ ·· ☆

JULY 2

Be Present

Be present right here, right now. Let the past live on in your memory and trust that the future will unfold naturally. This moment is the only one that matters, the only one that is real. It is in this moment that you are truly alive. Embrace it.

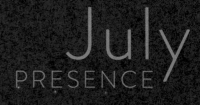

JULY 3

Cherish This Moment

It can be challenging to tune out your mind and be present in this moment. But realize that this version of you is fleeting. You will never again be exactly who or where you are right now. So slow down and immerse yourself within your current experience.

☆ ·· ☆

JULY 4

Just Be

Become aware of your presence. Sit with your thoughts, your feelings, and the sensations in your body. Find your breath. Let everything else fall away and, if only for a moment, allow yourself to just be.

JULY 5

Your Thoughts Are Visitors

Your thoughts and feelings are not your own. They are visitors, belonging to the universal mind. They are energy in motion, temporarily traveling through your vessel. Allow them to visit and then send them on their way.

☆ .... ☆

JULY 6

The Universe Speaks

The Universe speaks in subtleties and symbols. It is the feather floating beside you as you walk or the number you've already noticed at least three times today. The Universe is constantly guiding you. Are you listening?

JULY 7

Stillness Creates Clarity

Have you ever noticed that when you gaze into water, the more it moves the less you know what lies beneath the surface? The same phenomenon occurs within you. The busier your thoughts, the more you will struggle to see clearly. Let your thoughts settle like moonlight on water, and watch stillness appear.

☆ .... ☆

JULY 8

Every Moment Is New

Practice looking at everything with fresh eyes. Look at flowers, your lover, the stars in the sky as if you have never seen them before. Because this much is true: every moment is now, and every moment is new.

JULY 9

There Is Nothing to Fear

You are safe within your mind. Let go of your restless thoughts and tune in to your body. Unaddressed feelings are stored within you, wanting to be acknowledged and released. Breathe into them. Let them move through you. With every breath, you create peace. You are transforming darkness into light.

✩ .... ✩

JULY 10

Notice Expansiveness

Sit outside tonight if you can. Look around, noticing the vastness of space and sky. Now, with eyes closed, recall again the expansiveness. What do you notice? Is there a divide between you and the space around you, or is everything connected? Settle into this realm of slowness and curiosity.

JULY 11

Never Lose Your Wonder

There is magic all around you. This so-called reality you observe through your senses is one of many realities in this infinite Universe. Tune in to your inner child and see the world through their eyes. Look at everything as though you are seeing it for the first time.

☆ .... ☆

JULY 12

Soak in the Moon's Energy

Take a moment to go over to your window and look up at the Moon. If you can't see her, close your eyes and use your imagination. Feel her stillness and the warmth of her glow. Soak in her gentle energy and allow her to remind you of the beauty of this moment.

JULY 13

Let the Earth Hold You

Sit quietly and draw your attention to your body. Release
any tension you're carrying and allow yourself to gently
sink into the ground below you. Keep sinking deeper and
deeper. The deeper you sink, the more relaxed you will
feel, and the more you will merge with the earth and with
this moment.

☆ ·· ☆

JULY 14

Silence Is Not Empty

Silence is full of answers. It is the birthplace of all creation. It
is the home of infinite possibility. It is the truth underneath
the noise. Listen to silence and you will learn the secrets
of the Universe.

JULY 15

Feel into Your Soul

Humans rely heavily on the five senses to make judgments and decisions. But your perception may be obscuring the truth. The senses are only one of many ways to gather information, and the outside world is only one of many realities that exist in this Universe. Close your eyes and look inside. Only then will your truth appear.

☆ ⋯⋯⋯⋯⋯⋯⋯⋯⋯⋯⋯⋯⋯⋯⋯ ☆

JULY 16

You Are Not Your Thoughts

The voices in your head are not you. You are the awareness behind the thoughts, the one observing your own mind. Your thoughts only matter if you give them power. You decide which thoughts to feed and which ones to release.

JULY 17

Your Body Is Wise

Draw your attention inward. Focus on the sensations you
are experiencing in this moment. Notice any tightness or
tension. Bring awareness to any messages that don't carry
words. Listen to the deep wisdom that lies within your body.

☆ .... ☆

JULY 18

Listen to Your Feelings

Your emotions are trying to communicate with you. Jealousy
shows you where you still have room to love yourself more.
Fear shows you where you need to take a step outside your
comfort zone. Your feelings are your guides.

JULY 19

Find Magic in the Ordinary

Some days you are standing on top of the tallest mountain. But most days are ordinary. Thrilling moments come and go like fireflies, and you are left with the simple, small things of daily life. Give these moments meaning.

☆ .... ☆

JULY 20

Every Breath Is a Rebirth

You are cocreating with the Universe in every moment. Every breath you take is a chance for a rebirth, an opportunity to embrace your highest self and to embody unconditional love. Never take this moment for granted.

JULY 21

Consider a New Perspective

Is your mind holding you back? Are you keeping yourself from seeing someone or something in a fresh, new light? There are several ways to view any given situation. Sometimes all you need is a change in perspective.

☆ .... ☆

JULY 22

Don't Miss the Present

The mind loves to make you believe that your thoughts deserve your full, undivided attention. But the more you focus on your thoughts, the more you miss the present. Play some soft music, gaze into a candle flame, or focus on your breath. Your thoughts will be okay without you.

☆ .... ☆

JULY 23

Be with Yourself

Try for a moment to just be still. Breathe in and out. Feel the gravity and weight of your body as you sit. Remind yourself that it's okay to do nothing. Just be with yourself. It's enough to simply exist, exactly as you are in this moment.

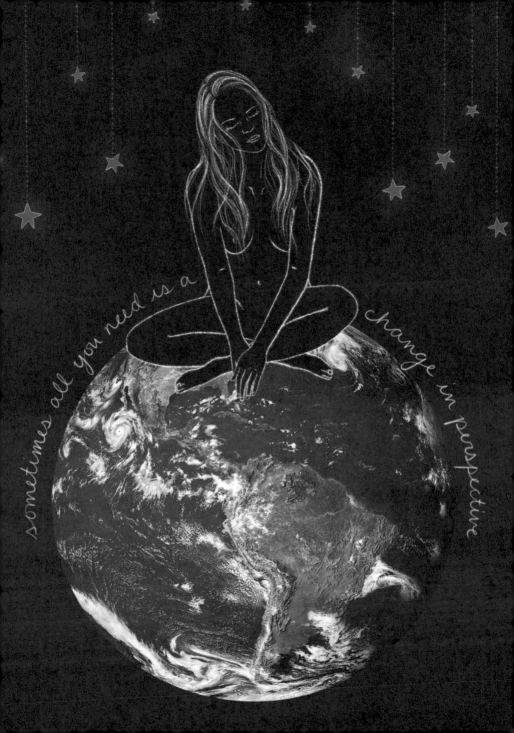

JULY 24

Awareness Is Power

The quieter you become, the more you develop the ability to see yourself from an outside perspective. This perspective allows you to detach, to observe your mind without judgment, and to become aware of harmful and unproductive patterns so that you can heal and grow.

☆ .... ☆

JULY 25

Presence Takes Practice

The mind loves to entertain itself. It finds the outside world endlessly fascinating. So, when you bring your attention inward, you may feel distracted, frustrated, or restless. Remind yourself of your personal motivations for meditating and remember that everything takes practice.

JULY 26

Stretch Your Body, Stretch Your Mind

Instead of meditating in a stoic position tonight, move your body. Notice where you feel tense and stretch those areas. Make gentle circles with your head; roll your shoulders forward and backward. When you release tension from your physical body, your mind relaxes, too.

✩ ·· ✩

JULY 27

Empty Your Mind

Imagine your thoughts as clouds gently floating away until the sky in your mind's eye is clear and blue. There is no thought so important that it cannot be reflected on later.

JULY 28

Use Your Imagination

Have you ever experienced being underwater? Imagine
yourself there now, beneath the surface. Keep breathing,
but notice the change in gravity, and feel how time seems
to slow down. Relax and let the water hold you. Remember
your imagination is here for you, anytime you need.

✩ .... ✩

JULY 29

Bring in Awareness

Between action and reaction lives a sacred pause, a
fleeting moment where time stops and you get to choose
how you handle the situation. Pause. Feel. Breathe, and
empower yourself to choose the higher path.

JULY 30

Listen

Your ego lives in your mind and wants to keep you comfortable and safe. Your soul contains your authenticity and wants to set you free. Presence is a mediator between these two parts of you. Tune in to this now moment and listen for the truth.

☆ ·· ☆

JULY 31

It's All About the Journey

Live for the current moment, not for the next moment. Do not get so caught up in working toward the future that you forget to be here in the present. There is no ultimate destination in life. The beauty, joy, and growth is in the journey itself.

AUGUST 1

Breathe

Your body is communicating with you right now—are you listening? That tension you're holding—lean in. Feel what is coming up for you. Breathe. Your body wants you to trust its guidance. It wants you to know that you are safe to feel.

☆ .... ☆

AUGUST 2

Trust the Unfolding

How often have you tried to control the outcome of something? How much anxiety have you battled in search of an "answer"? The path may not unfold in the way you plan or imagine, but that doesn't make it any less magnificent.

August
TRUST

AUGUST 3

Surrender

Surrendering to the Universe means not spending your energy controlling or fighting the powerful forces that be. It means believing in something greater than the struggle of your current situation. It is an act of courage and trust. Let yourself surrender.

☆ ·· ☆

AUGUST 4

Clarity Will Come

When you are torn between different possible paths, remember that clarity cannot be found through an anxious mind. The answer will come through quiet self-reflection or through your intuition. You may know what you need to do, even if you can't explain why. Either way, trust that clarity will come.

AUGUST 5

Rejection Is Redirection

What feels like rejection is actually redirection. The Universe is clearing space to make room for something or someone far more suited to your soul. You may not see it now, but someday you will. What's meant for you will not pass you by.

✧ ·· ✧

AUGUST 6

New Doors Will Open

Setting boundaries may seem limiting, but it only limits that which does not resonate with you. Boundaries make way for new opportunities, new relationships, and new growth. You never know what doors will open when you close the ones that are not meant for you.

AUGUST 7

Your Intuition Will Guide You

When you want to take a risk or to try something new, you will know when you are ready. Not because you feel fearless or have complete trust and confidence, but because you know. You just know, and that is all the reason you need. Your intuition will not lead you astray.

☆ ··· ☆

AUGUST 8

Follow Your Visions

Your visions are not in vain. Connect with the earth and stay grounded but know that your idealism is not foolish. Your visions come to you for a reason. They are guiding you toward your purpose. Follow them.

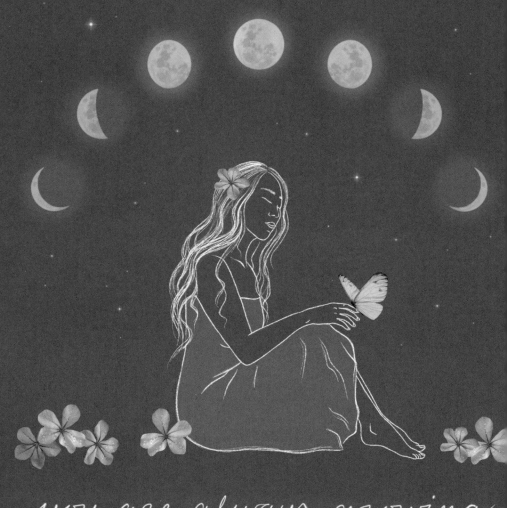

you are always growing

even when you don't feel it

AUGUST 9

Open Your Mind

It's time to let go of the illusion of control. Life doesn't always go according to plan, but that doesn't mean things aren't working out. Loosen your grip. Open your mind to the idea that your path may be unfolding in exactly the way it is meant to.

☆ ⋯⋯⋯⋯⋯⋯⋯⋯⋯⋯⋯⋯⋯⋯⋯ ☆

AUGUST 10

The Unknown Is Sacred

There is something sacred about not knowing the future, about understanding that you and the Universe will cocreate so much learning, growth, and healing, but not knowing the details. Recognize the wonder that lies in the mystery of the unknown.

☆ ⋯⋯⋯⋯⋯⋯⋯⋯⋯⋯⋯⋯⋯⋯⋯ ☆

AUGUST 11

You Are Always Growing

You are always transforming, even when you don't feel it. Sometimes you might believe you are moving backward when actually you are being given an opportunity to strengthen your ability to navigate the natural twists and turns of life. Dive in and trust the process.

AUGUST 12

Everything Works Out

There is no reason to agonize over choices or decisions. There is no right or wrong when your heart and intentions are pure. Everything has a way of working out, even when you don't yet see how.

☆ .... ☆

AUGUST 13

Find Order in Chaos

Outer space may seem overwhelming and out of control, but order does exist in the Universe. Stars can be mapped, planets rotate in trackable patterns, even meteor showers can be predicted. If such massive celestial bodies and events are not random, then might there be order to the events in your life, too?

AUGUST 14

You Are Held

The Universe has existed for billions of years. It is older and wiser than the human mind can comprehend. Trust that you are always held in the hands of the Universe, and that you are safe to explore what lies on the other side of fear.

☆ .... ☆

AUGUST 15

Lean In Deeper

Your ego may think it knows what's best for you, but may instead be blocking your connection with your soul. Check in with your emotions. Have you been acting out of fear or out of love? Can you let yourself lean deeper into trust?

AUGUST 16

Share Your Medicine

The things that light you up are not random. They are signs from the Universe, highlighting your potential and guiding you toward your greater purpose. Your heart, creativity and talents are medicine that can help heal, nurture, and inspire others. Follow the light.

✩ .... ✩

AUGUST 17

Every Path Brings Value

The choices in this life are endless. Do not waste time fretting over which path to follow. Any path you choose can bring you value and growth. Follow your heart and choose from a place of trust. The view from every mountain is magnificent.

AUGUST 18

You Are Abundant

Every day, your thoughts are filtered through your perceptions, and decisions are made based on those perceptions. Perceive yourself as capable, and you will be. Believe you are abundant, and you will be. Your internal beliefs will always be reflected in your external world.

☆ ·· ☆

AUGUST 19

Change Is Natural

Dragonflies begin as water nymphs, living under water before bursting through the surface and growing wings. Changing one's environment must be challenging, but can you imagine the discomfort of trying to fly under water? As difficult as it may be, trust that change is for your highest good.

AUGUST 20

You Are Not Lost

You are never truly lost. When you feel this way, what you might be feeling is the confusing and uncomfortable process of release. You are shedding your skin, releasing everything you carried with you before you remembered who you are.

☆ .... ☆

AUGUST 21

Your Soul Knows the Way

Listen to that still, quiet whisper of wisdom within you. Trust your inner guidance. No one but you can know what is best for you. This is your life, and you are the captain. Follow your soul and trust that it knows the way.

AUGUST 22

You Are Supported

There isn't always a "right time" to do something. Sometimes it's your doubt that holds you back. Sometimes you have to jump before you see the net. You have to believe in yourself and believe that the Universe is always there to support you.

☆ .... ☆

AUGUST 23

Let Life Surprise You

You think you know what you want. You think you know how you want your life to unfold. But do you really? Haven't some of the most beautiful moments, the most beautiful people you've met, been serendipitous? Let life take you through unexpected turns and see where they lead you.

AUGUST 24

Trust Yourself

When you don't know which way to turn, go inward. Acknowledge your doubts, fears, and insecurities. Remember, there is no wrong decision. Feel what you need to feel. Let go and trust that you will make the best decision for yourself.

✧ ·· ✧

AUGUST 25

Ease Your Mind

Meditate tonight with only candlelight. Turn off any artificial lights, and gently gaze into the candle's flame, making it your sole focus. If your eyes grow tired, close them and imagine the flame in your mind's eye. This practice will ease your wandering mind and calm your spirit.

AUGUST 26

Protect Your Energy

Be careful how you spend your energy. Not all actions require a reaction, and not all people will be receptive to your perspectives. Sometimes the most loving thing you can do is to create space between yourself and another person or situation. Trust your inner guidance.

☆ .... ☆

AUGUST 27

Everything Is Working Out

Your mind wants to figure everything out. To pick up pieces of the past, examine anxieties and fears, and try to make sense of it all. But the Universe works in mysterious ways. Have faith that you will end up exactly where you need to be.

AUGUST 28

You Are Being Guided

When you feel you are floating aimlessly with no direction or purpose, know that the Universe has not forgotten you. You may not feel it to be true right now, but someday you will look back and see that you were being guided all along.

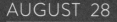

AUGUST 29

Release Your Past

Become aware of old stories attaching you to the past. These narratives prevent you from being present with who you are now and from blossoming into your future self. Do not carry your past with you. Trust that you are safe to let go.

AUGUST 30

Remain Open

Be mindful of expectation. When you are fixed to one particular path, you close yourself off to all other possibilities. Open yourself up. The Universe may have something in store for you that surpasses what you've imagined for yourself.

☆ .... ☆

AUGUST 31

Trust Time

Trust that what's meant to come into your life will come, and what's meant to go will go. There is nothing wrong with the path you have traveled so far, and nothing missing from your life in this moment. Trust the timing of your life.

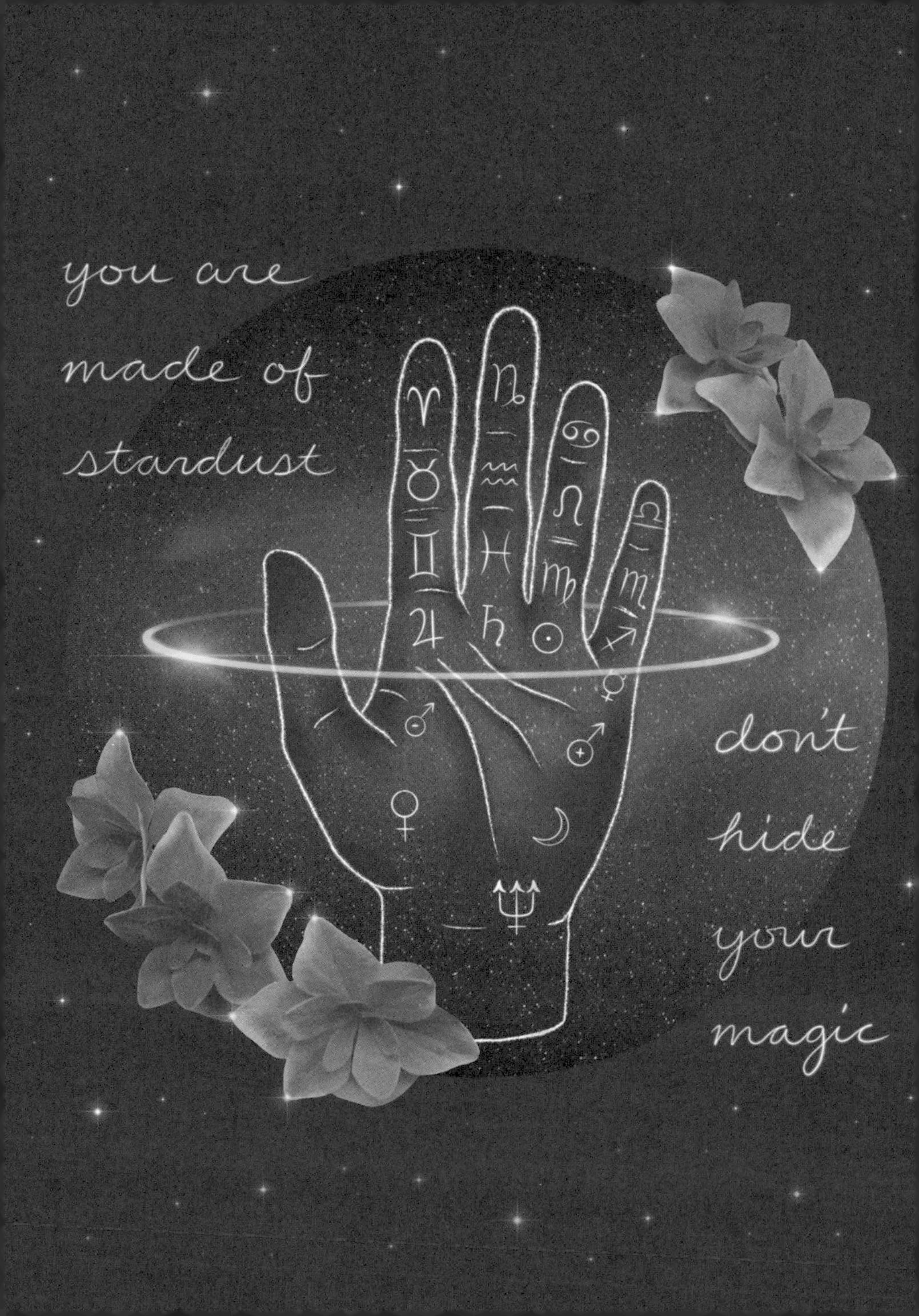
you are
made of
stardust
don't
hide
your
magic

September
COURAGE

SEPTEMBER 1

Don't Hide Your Magic

There is magic pulsing through your veins. You are an energetic being of light, the elements in your body created from stardust bound together with skin and bones and earth. There is nothing ordinary about you. Don't hide away the magic you hold.

SEPTEMBER 2

No More Playing Small

Everything on this planet plays an integral role in the Universe. And you, being a creation of the Universe, are no exception. No one benefits when you shrink yourself and play small. Dare to take up space.

✩ .... ✩

SEPTEMBER 3

Be like a Tree

When leaves begin to lose their color and fall to the ground, the tree does not cower away. Instead, it boldly prepares for the next phase of life. Sit now like a tree, straight and tall, and remind yourself you have the courage to face whatever may come your way.

SEPTEMBER 4

Take the Risk

It's not about being fearless. It's not about ridding yourself of this very normal, very human emotion. It's about feeling fear and not letting it hold you back. It's about taking the risk despite the fear. You can be afraid and still be brave.

☆ .... ☆

SEPTEMBER 5

It's Okay to Feel Lost

You may feel uncertain about your path in life, but being lost means you had the courage to go out seeking in the first place. Be proud of the times you've stepped out of your comfort zone and explored new opportunities. Keep being brave. Sometimes it takes getting lost to find yourself again.

SEPTEMBER 6

Look Within

People love to offer advice. But no one knows you better than you, and no one can tell you how best to live your life. Look inside rather than outside to discover your own answers, perspectives, and beliefs. And have the courage to express what you find.

☆ ·· ☆

SEPTEMBER 7

Listen to Your Soul

When you begin facing your fears, your mind will conjure up all sorts of false ideas about you not being capable enough, strong enough, or worthy enough. Your ego wants to protect you. But remember that your soul knows better.

SEPTEMBER 8

Keep Sharing Your Light

There is no such thing as normal. Normal is a word used to describe those afraid to be themselves. Everyone is unique, and everyone is designed to share their gifts with the world. Be proud of yourself for being brave enough to shine.

☆ ···································· ☆

SEPTEMBER 9

You Are Nature

Something wild is calling you home. There is ancient wisdom deep within your DNA, reminding you of your true essence. You are nature, and you intuitively know who you are and how to move through this life.

SEPTEMBER 10

Live Your Truth

The more you are you, the more you are free. There will always be external limitations, but true freedom comes from within. It comes from knowing that you are the sole authority of your life and being brave enough to live your truth.

☆ ⋯⋯⋯⋯⋯⋯⋯⋯⋯⋯⋯⋯⋯⋯⋯ ☆

SEPTEMBER 11

Release Your Past Self

You cannot embrace or express your most authentic self without first releasing what binds you to the past. Have the courage to let go of who you thought you were to make room for who you are becoming.

have the
courage
to let go
of who you
thought you
were
to make room
for who
you are
becoming

SEPTEMBER 12

It's Okay

It's okay to be scared. It's okay to be afraid of being judged and misunderstood. It's okay to be afraid of change. It's okay to be afraid of your own shadow. It's okay. It's all okay.

✩ ·· ✩

SEPTEMBER 13

Plant Yourself in New Soil

There is comfort in a predictable life lived inside the confines of your comfort zone. The path is certain and safe. But no flowers grow there. Be brave enough to step outside the box and plant yourself in new soil.

SEPTEMBER 14

Face Your Shadows

The Universe is your mirror. The light and dark in the world reflect the light and dark within you. When you're struggling, summon the courage to face the shadows. You may be surprised to find that they lead you to the light.

☆ ·· ☆

SEPTEMBER 15

Start Walking

You don't need to see a clear path in front of you in order to begin. All you need is a vision in your heart and a drive to create. Start walking and the path will appear.

SEPTEMBER 16

Take a Chance

Take a chance on yourself. Focus your time and energy on what makes you feel alive. You are your greatest investment, and it is time to do more than merely survive. It is time to thrive.

☆ .... ☆

SEPTEMBER 17

Take Responsibility

Take responsibility for yourself. This does not mean carrying regret, guilt, or shame. It means realizing that there are shadows you are holding on to and acknowledging that you may project them on to others sometimes. Instead of denying or repressing your emotions, summon the courage to feel, embrace, and integrate.

SEPTEMBER 18

Embrace Your Fears

Welcome your doubts and fears. When you no longer allow these feelings to hold power over you, you naturally create space for your true self to emerge. You begin to fully embody the beauty, freedom, and uniqueness that is you. And because you are authentically, unapologetically yourself, you help others gain the courage to be themselves, too.

☆ .... ☆

SEPTEMBER 19

Listen to the Universe

The Universe wants the best for you. It knows what you need to grow and heal, and it will send you the same message repeatedly, in all manner of ways, until you have the courage to listen.

SEPTEMBER 20

You Are Undefinable

Your life story is valuable, but it doesn't define you. You are so much more than your experiences. You are a free spirit whose soul cannot be labeled or contained. Strip away anything that holds you down, and step into your limitless, multidimensional self.

☆ .... ☆

SEPTEMBER 21

Keep Shining

Sometimes your light will confuse or aggravate others. They may judge, reject, or deeply misunderstand you. They may even blame you for blinding them. But it is not your fault they are afraid to look within. Their fear is not yours to carry.

☆ .... ☆

SEPTEMBER 22

Look Deeper

You are likely not procrastinating simply out of laziness. There is a deeper meaning underneath the resistance you feel. Are you putting something off because you feel incompetent, unworthy, or afraid? Sit with your resistance for a while and you might find your answer.

SEPTEMBER 23

Take Responsibility

Take responsibility for yourself. This does not mean carrying regret, guilt, or shame. It means realizing that there are shadows you are holding on to and acknowledging that you may project them on to others sometimes. Instead of denying or repressing your emotions, summon the courage to feel, embrace, and integrate.

☆ .... ☆

SEPTEMBER 24

Imagine You Are the Moon

You are soft and gentle yet powerful and bright like the Moon. You are steady and unwavering no matter the darkness around you. You trust nature and the rhythms of life. And you radiate in whatever way feels right.

SEPTEMBER 25

You Are a Seed

Close your eyes and imagine a seed deep within the earth. The soil is cold and dark, and the seed feels afraid. Now, imagine you are that seed. Let the emotion move through your body. Expose yourself to the darkness. And then realize there is nothing to fear because you have not been buried: you have been planted.

☆ .... ☆

SEPTEMBER 26

Courage Comes in Many Forms

Courage often means facing fear by taking action. But sometimes, courage asks for inaction. There is bravery in yielding your control and being receptive to what the Universe wants to give you. Reflect on your current situation and ask yourself which type of courage you currently need.

SEPTEMBER 27

The Universe Rewards the Brave

Birds are not born with the ability to fly. Flying requires practice and courage. They must be brave enough to jump off the branch and likely fall down a good handful of times. But their courage is not in vain. Those who take a leap of faith are always rewarded.

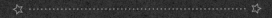

SEPTEMBER 28

See Where You Might Go

A clear path ahead is tempting to follow. It appears welcoming in its comfort and security. But the path has already been traveled. You know it isn't yours. So, turn around. Take one step at a time. See where you might go.

SEPTEMBER 29

Fear Is a Sign

Fear does not come to harm you. Often it arrives to illuminate whatever it is you want but are afraid of. Lean into the fear. Let it move through you. On the other side of fear is love and freedom.

☆ .... ☆

SEPTEMBER 30

Summon the Courage

You cannot go through the same motions every day, carrying around the same old habits and mind-set, and expect growth. Change comes from breaking patterns, from trying something new. You will never know your full potential if you do not summon the courage to live the life you've always dreamed of living.

OCTOBER 1

Find Your Way Back Home

Go easy on yourself. Take your time. You are shedding outgrown layers of yourself. You are releasing the weight of your past, the opinions of others, and the beliefs and patterns that no longer serve you. You are coming home to yourself.

☆ .... ☆

OCTOBER 2

There Are No Bad Emotions

Society labels certain emotions as "positive" and others as "negative." But just because an emotion is painful or uncomfortable does not make it bad. These feelings are natural and necessary. They pave a path for healing.

October

HEALING

OCTOBER 3

Listen and Let Go

Your body intuitively knows how to heal itself. There is ancient wisdom hidden deep within your bones, more intelligent even than your mind and your heart. All you need to do is listen. Listen and let go of all that needs to be released.

☆ .... ☆

OCTOBER 4

Love Your Past Self

Do not discount your past self. Do not look down on them or shame them for their behaviors. Forgive them. Understand them. Love them and be proud of them. Without them you wouldn't be who you are today.

OCTOBER 5

The Rain Is Necessary

You cannot expect to feel joy in every moment. But even in the dark, you can still remind yourself that the rain is necessary for the plants to grow. You can still appreciate the lessons that every season brings.

✫ ·· ✫

OCTOBER 6

Embrace the Journey

Polarity is the way of the Universe. Light cannot exist without darkness. There is no joy without pain, and no pain without joy. Whatever you are going through is natural. You are simply experiencing what it means to be human. Embrace where you are on your journey.

OCTOBER 7

Make Peace with Being Misunderstood

Make peace with the truth that many will not see or understand you. Find love and belonging first within yourself, and the people meant for you will arrive in your life when they are meant to.

☆ ·· ☆

OCTOBER 8

Appreciate the Darkness

The dark and light are forever intertwined. They dance together everywhere, from the night sky to the depths of your being. Appreciate the darkness, for without it you wouldn't be able to see the light.

OCTOBER 9

Nurture Your Inner Child

Take this time to connect with your inner child. Listen to whatever it is they need, the pain they want you to acknowledge, the forgiveness they are seeking. Maybe they want to connect with curiosity and creativity, to make more room for play and exploration. Listen without judgment, and welcome all that comes.

✩ ·· ✩

OCTOBER 10

Listen to Your Body

When your body feels tight and restricted, it is holding on to something that needs to be released. Tension is your body's way of communicating with you that there is healing work needing to be done in this moment. Pay attention and listen.

OCTOBER 11

Your Sensitivity Is a Gift

Sensitivity is not a weakness. It is your sensitivity that connects you with your emotions and opens a pathway for healing. It is your sensitivity that allows you to experience a life of depth and meaning, and to have deep compassion for others as well.

☆ .... ☆

OCTOBER 12

Love Is the Only Way

The more you love yourself, the more you will love others. You may not love everyone's opinions and actions, but you will see how all humans have the same needs for acceptance, safety, and peace. No matter someone's experiences, your heart will reach out to them, because even the unkindest need love, and love is the only path to healing.

OCTOBER 13

Tune In to Your Breath

Tune in to your breath. Become aware of the rise and fall of your body as you inhale and exhale. Allow yourself to notice whatever thoughts and feelings come up for you. Keep breathing and remind yourself that everything is temporary. Let this moment be what it is.

☆ .... ☆

OCTOBER 14

Accept All of You

Your being contains many aspects. Sometimes you will feel integrated and whole, and other times you will feel at war within yourself. But all parts of you, especially the seemingly most conflicting, are valid and valuable. Embrace all of you.

OCTOBER 15

You Are Not Alone

Healing is an inside job. No teacher, guide, parent, or friend can do it for you. But that doesn't mean you can't seek support. There is strength in asking for help. Remember, you are not alone.

☆ .... ☆

OCTOBER 16

Darkness Births Light

Have you noticed that the darker the sky, the more clearly the stars appear? The same happens within you. The more difficult and painful your thoughts and emotions become, the more potential there is for gratitude and love to emerge. The deeper the darkness, the brighter the light.

OCTOBER 17

Choose to Be Grateful

Every situation brings an opportunity for empowerment.
No matter how dark or painful the experience, you can
always choose to be grateful for the lessons you've learned
and for the strength you've discovered within yourself that
you never knew you had.

☆ ·· ☆

OCTOBER 18

Let Your Emotions Help You

Your emotions do not belong to your body. They are not
stuck inside you. It is safe to let them stay for a while.
They need you to fulfill their purpose, just as you need
them to fulfill yours. Let them help you heal.

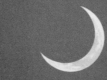

OCTOBER 19

Keep Your Heart Open

In the midst of confusion and stress, it is difficult to clear your mind. What you are going through may feel unnecessary and unfair. But if you make room in your heart for the possibility that clarity can be found, you open up a space where peace and healing can take place.

✧ ⋯⋯⋯⋯⋯⋯⋯⋯⋯⋯⋯⋯⋯⋯⋯⋯⋯ ✧

OCTOBER 20

Let Yourself Feel

Sometimes it's simply too hard to look at the bright side. In times like these, it's okay to sit with yourself in the dark for as long as you need. Give yourself permission to feel everything. You are resilient, and you will be okay.

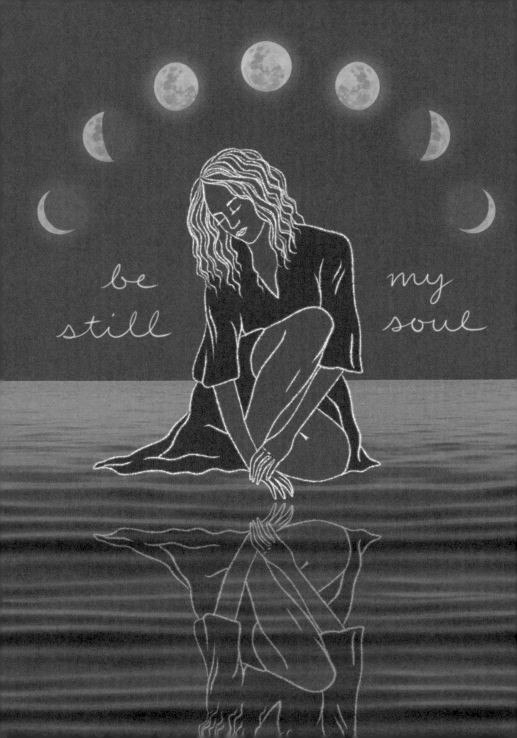

OCTOBER 21

Be Still

Only when you are still can you see clearly. Only when you tune out the voices within and around you can you tune in to the stillness that resides within your body and heart. Only when you truly feel what needs to be felt can you allow yourself to heal.

☆ ·· ☆

OCTOBER 22

You Are an Alchemist

Think of the times your body has healed itself from cuts and bruises. Remember when you thought your heart would never mend, but it did. You have overcome every difficult day. And here you are, once again alchemizing fear and pain into faith and strength.

☆ ·· ☆

OCTOBER 23

Stress Is a Sign

Stress is a sign that it's time to look within. It shows up not to break you down, but to guide you toward where you most need to heal. Do not ignore or run from it. Bring the emotion into focus. You need to feel in order to heal.

OCTOBER 24

Welcome Your Contradictions

You are full of beautiful contradictions. You are both aggressive and gentle, cynical and hopeful, fire and water. You are simple, subtle, and complex. Allow all parts of you. All are valid. Your contradictions make you whole.

☆ .... ☆

OCTOBER 25

Healing Happens Slowly

When you ignore, repress, or run from something, it will keep coming back. Even when you bravely face your feelings, they may not be gone forever. Some wounds run deep, and some patterns take years to unravel. Give yourself time.

OCTOBER 26

Do Not Blame Others

Do not blame others for your triggers. The things that create turbulence within you are your responsibility, and they will only keep returning if you push them away. So let them move through you. Breathe through the feelings, cry them out, do whatever sets them free. This is how you can start to work on healing.

☆ .... ☆

OCTOBER 27

Distractions Delay Healing

Distractions only delay the inner work that needs to be done. Challenges always return when they are not addressed. Simply by sitting here tonight, by putting down your phone and settling into quiet self-reflection, you have already opened the pathway to healing.

OCTOBER 28

Your Body Knows

Healing doesn't happen in a steady, forward motion. It's normal to find yourself working through something you thought was behind you. But constantly thinking about your struggles may not ease your pain. Pain is stored in the body and therefore can be healed through the body. Tune in and notice the wisdom within.

✩ ⋯⋯⋯⋯⋯⋯⋯⋯⋯⋯⋯⋯⋯⋯⋯⋯ ✩

OCTOBER 29

Your Feelings Are Guides

Jealousy is not inherently bad. When you feel jealous of another person, your feelings are guiding you toward where you feel incapable, unworthy, or incomplete. You are being shown where there is room to heal. Come back to yourself. Give yourself grace and love.

OCTOBER 30

You Can't Rush Your Healing

Healing happens at its own pace. Sometimes you think you've moved on and then your pain knocks back on your door, asking to be seen again. Take your time. Be gentle with yourself.

☆ .... ☆

OCTOBER 31

Heal Yourself, Heal the World

Separation is an illusion. Every thought and emotion you have, every action you take, reverberates throughout the Universe. The more care and love you give yourself, the more love will radiate onto others. When you begin to heal yourself, you begin to heal the world.

NOVEMBER 1

Dive into the Depths

It is natural to fear the darkness. But in the depths of your consciousness lies massive potential for healing and growth. It is in the places where you are afraid and resistant to look that you will find magic.

☆ ⋯⋯⋯⋯⋯⋯⋯⋯⋯⋯⋯⋯⋯⋯⋯⋯ ☆

NOVEMBER 2

Water Your Mind

The mind is a powerful thing. Change your mind-set and your life will change, too. The external is a reflection of your internal world. There is no separation. Water your mind with uplifting thoughts and the world around you will blossom.

November
TRANSFORMATION

NOVEMBER 3

The Moon Takes Her Time

Every month, the Moon slowly and steadily transforms herself from dark to light and back again. Nature cannot rush her rhythms, nor should she. Every phase is a necessary part of the cycle. Take after the Moon and be patient with yourself as you travel along your ever-changing journey.

☆ .... ☆

NOVEMBER 4

Embrace the Process

Whatever you are currently going through is preparing you to meet the next version of yourself. When you embrace the process and allow whatever comes up for you, you activate your highest time line. You open the doorway to your highest potential.

NOVEMBER 5

Flow with Change

Acknowledge the uncomfortable feelings that arise when facing the unknown. In a world that is ever-evolving, change is the only constant. The more you practice sitting with discomfort, the more you will be able to flow with whatever changes come your way.

☆ ·· ☆

NOVEMBER 6

Keep Shedding Your Skin

You will outgrow yourself over and over again. You will shed your skin so many times that you no longer recognize the person you used to be. Do not let others get in the way of you recreating yourself as many times as you need.

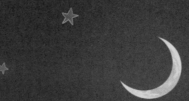

NOVEMBER 7

Thoughts Can Be Unlearned

The voice of the inner critic is not yours. Thoughts come from the external and are internalized as your own. You were not born with them—you learned them. Remember this when troubling thoughts enter your mind. The remembrance will lessen their power so they can be unlearned.

☆ ·· ☆

NOVEMBER 8

You Are Enveloped in Love

Visualize a ball of white light above your head. The sphere is warm and alive with energy. It represents the love of the Universe. Now take a deep breath in and, as you exhale, imagine the light slowly washing over you, melting away tension, and enveloping you with soft, gentle warmth.

NOVEMBER 9

Your Journey Is Worth It

The spiritual journey is not easy. It requires patience, practice, and courage. But the challenge is precisely what makes the journey so rewarding. Trust that the work you put in will be worth the joy, peace, and freedom that await you on the other side. Your spiritual journey is worth the challenge.

☆ .... ☆

NOVEMBER 10

Be Patient with Yourself

The caterpillar does not become the butterfly overnight. The transition from here to there is scary, challenging, and uncomfortable. Give yourself time to grow your wings. Be patient with yourself and with who you are becoming.

NOVEMBER 11

Open Mind, Open Heart

Judgment has its time and place. But observation holds
a much higher vibration. Observation opens your mind
and your heart. When you feel judgment creep in, observe
what you are feeling, what you are "judging." This gives
you an opportunity to learn and grow, to broaden your
perspective and deepen your compassion.

☆ .... ☆

NOVEMBER 12

Recreate Yourself

The human body renews its cells every seven to ten years.
Your body is continuously transforming. Isn't it only natural,
then, that your mind is always changing, too? Do not let
others' expectations or your own self-limiting beliefs keep
you stuck. Recreate yourself as often as you please.

NOVEMBER 13

Allow Change

Fighting that which is not within your control will only cause you suffering. When the wind is harsh and cold, when it burns your face and brings tears to your eyes, carry on. Know it will settle soon. And when the wind is at your back, be grateful.

☆ .... ☆

NOVEMBER 14

Honor Your Journey

After a transformation, your energy vibrates at a different rate than it used to and is no longer a vibrational match with your former self. The people and things you once held dear may no longer resonate with you. It's okay to move on. Honor where you are on your journey.

NOVEMBER 15

Change Is Okay

Those who wish for you to stay the same are struggling with change themselves, or fear that they will lose you. Remember that relationships come and go, but your relationship with yourself is forever. It's okay to put your needs first.

☆ .... ☆

NOVEMBER 16

Choose Differently

When turbulence arises between you and another person, rather than projecting your feelings onto them, bring in awareness. Pause for a moment before reacting. Realize that you always have the power to choose differently.

NOVEMBER 17

Accept Yourself

You cannot guilt or shame yourself into change. Rather, these emotions will distance you from yourself and from love. Love is acceptance. It is only when you accept yourself unconditionally, in all your complicated, messy, wonderful humanness, that you can begin to change.

✧ ⋯⋯⋯⋯⋯⋯⋯⋯⋯⋯⋯⋯⋯⋯⋯⋯ ✧

NOVEMBER 18

Embrace Discomfort

Change is not always comfortable. The cocoon is not spacious. But it's where you learn the most about yourself, where you become most acquainted with the depths of your soul. Embrace the darkness and the quiet. Without the chrysalis there would be no butterflies.

NOVEMBER 19

Choose Love

You may not have control over everything that happens in life, but you always have control over your response. You have the choice to react with fear and judgment or to take the higher road of forgiveness, understanding, and love.

☆ .... ☆

NOVEMBER 20

Change Begins Within

Change happens from the inside out. Look inside. Be brave enough to see every part of you. Know that simply by having the courage to acknowledge it all, and to feel it all, you allow for transformation to begin.

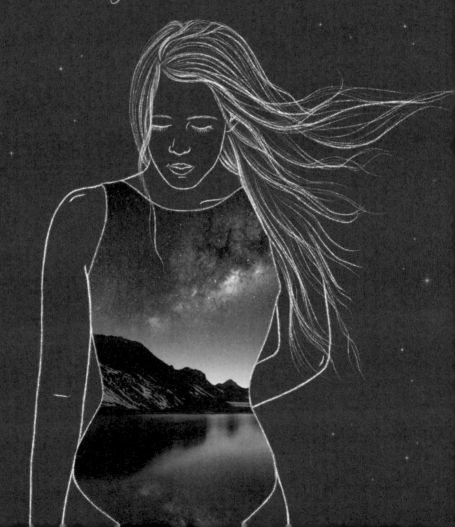

guided by the compass
of my inner universe

NOVEMBER 21

You Are Always Guided

Wherever you go, you are guided by the compass of your inner world. Empower yourself to be the captain of your own life. You will not lead yourself astray.

☆ ·· ☆

NOVEMBER 22

Do What Feels Right

When people say, "Follow your heart," they mean, "Do what feels right." Listen to that sense of knowingness that may not make sense at all. Logic is far from the deepest source of wisdom. Follow the voice that doesn't speak—the voice of your soul.

NOVEMBER 23

Energy Can Change Form

Energy cannot be created or destroyed; it can only change form. Remember this as you sit here, wishing to transition into a calmer state of being. Transform your thoughts and feelings by gently saying to yourself, "I am not anxiety; I am peace. I am not stress; I am ease."

NOVEMBER 24

You Will Adjust

What is healthy might not feel good at first. If you are accustomed to anxiety, you may feel unsafe being at peace. If you are releasing a pattern of attracting toxic people, you may be uncomfortable when treated kindly. Give yourself time to adjust.

NOVEMBER 25

Take Back Your Power

What you fear is not the outcome of an undesirable situation, but rather the feelings that may result from it. You are afraid of feeling pain. However, your emotions can only control you if you give them the power to do so. Feel the fear and take back your power.

✩ ··· ✩

NOVEMBER 26

Outgrow Your Old Patterns

Sometimes the patterns that once served to keep you safe now keep you stuck. What makes your ego feel comfortable is usually not the route that holds the greatest potential for growth. Let yourself say goodbye to the old and create new pathways. You are ready.

NOVEMBER 27

You Are Learning

There is nothing wrong with any thought or emotion, or whatever experience you are going through. Remember that you are simply having a human experience. You are observing and learning and evolving. And you are right where you are supposed to be.

☆ ⋯⋯⋯⋯⋯⋯⋯⋯⋯⋯⋯⋯⋯⋯ ☆

NOVEMBER 28

Alchemize Your Feelings

You have the power to alchemize your feelings with your conscious awareness. Let go of your mind and tune in to your body. Breathe in the turbulence that moves within you, then breathe it out. Repeat as many times as you need, until the feelings fade.

NOVEMBER 29

Interpret Your Dreams

The conscious and subconscious mind communicate with one another while you sleep. Dreams often produce strange visions, but they might carry important insight into your current life situation. When you go to sleep tonight, ask yourself to remember your dreams, and in the morning, reflect on what you recall.

☆ .... ☆

NOVEMBER 30

Light the Way

When you explore the depths of your own soul, you open the door not only for your own transformation, but also for the transformation of others. When you alchemize your darkness into light, you pave a path for others to do the same.

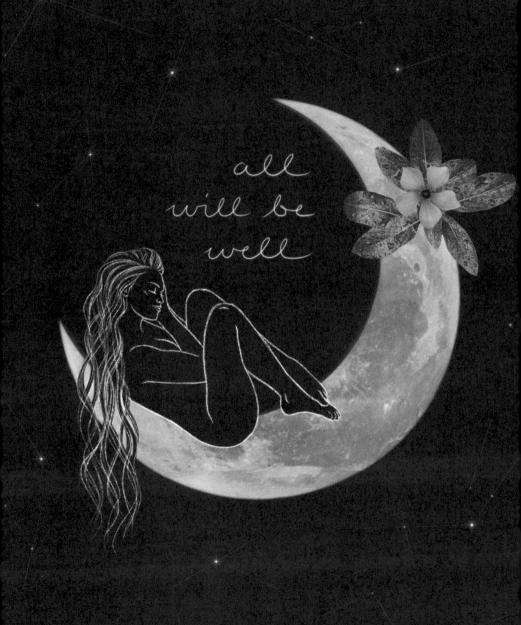

December
INNER PEACE

DECEMBER 1

All Will Be Well

The darkness is not to be feared. It is in the dark that you discover the ever-flowing well of peace that never leaves you. It is in the dark that you see the power of your own light and know that all will be well.

✦ ·· ✦

DECEMBER 2

Prioritize Your Peace

When you make peace a priority, decisions become clearer. The actions and reactions of others feel less personal. The overactive mind slows down, and challenging situations become easier to navigate. Life becomes simpler and, in turn, more beautiful.

DECEMBER 3

Recall the Sun

When sunlight shines on ice, the ice melts. It loses its hardness, surrendering to the warmth of the Sun's rays and allowing itself to soften. When you feel hardened by life's challenges, recall the Sun. Open yourself up so it can melt away your troubles.

☆ .... ☆

DECEMBER 4

Have No Regrets

Make peace with your past. When you look back, there may be many things you wish you had done differently. But there is no sense in looking back with regret. You've grown, and that's the point—that's what life is all about.

DECEMBER 5

Peace Is Your True Essence

Living peacefully does not mean ignoring your emotions. Rather, it means welcoming all feelings as a necessary part of life and allowing them to freely move through you. Peace is omnipresent and can always be found under every emotion. Peace is your natural state of being. It is your true essence.

☆ ⋯⋯⋯⋯⋯⋯⋯⋯⋯⋯⋯⋯⋯⋯⋯ ☆

DECEMBER 6

Boundaries Can Be Loving

Setting a boundary does not necessarily mean building a wall that blocks you from another person. A boundary can be created out of love. It is a way to show respect to yourself and the other person, allowing you both to learn and grow.

DECEMBER 7

Allow Yourself to Fail

There is no shame or loss in making mistakes. There is only learning and growth. Let yourself feel disappointed and discouraged but realize that failure is the only path to success. Mistakes lead you closer to where you're meant to go.

✩ ⋯⋯⋯⋯⋯⋯⋯⋯⋯⋯⋯⋯⋯⋯⋯ ✩

DECEMBER 8

Journal Your Thoughts

Keep some paper and a pen nearby while you meditate tonight. When a thought refuses to leave you alone, or you are reminded of something you need to do, write it down and then continue meditating. This simple act makes your mind feel important enough to quiet down and open space for stillness.

DECEMBER 9

Surround Yourself with Light

Peace is an inside job, but you are not separate from your environment. The outside world can drain you or it can light you up. Surround yourself with things and people who make you feel inspired.

☆ .... ☆

DECEMBER 10

Awaken to Oneness

The longer you sit in stillness, the more connected you will feel with everything around you. Your body is living, breathing energy. It is not separate from your surroundings. You are free and whole and one with everything in this Universe.

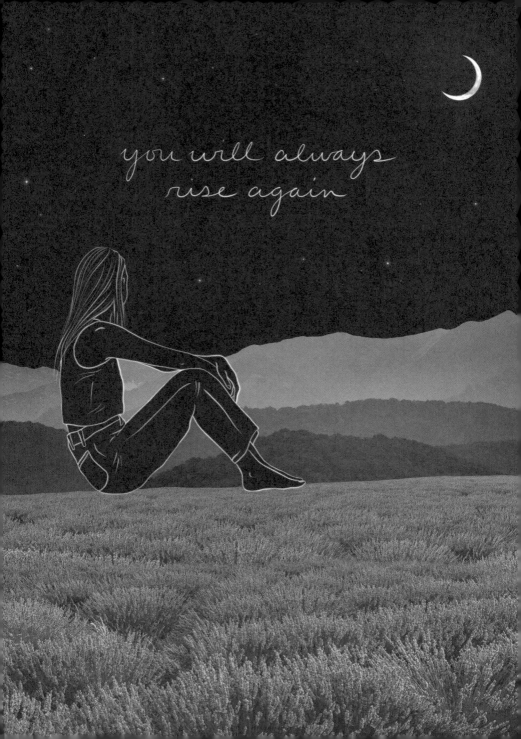

DECEMBER 11

You Will Always Rise Again

Evening turns to twilight, and twilight to dawn. Nature is always in flux, never stagnant, and your life flows in the same way. When your soul needs soothing, remember that even the darkest night becomes day.

☆ .... ☆

DECEMBER 12

Be like an Owl

Owls have long been considered a symbol of wisdom. With their powerful sense of sight, they see what most others cannot. The owl takes advantage of the night, and so can you. Sit in full darkness tonight, and tune in to your senses. What new insights can you find in the stillness of the night?

DECEMBER 13

Your Energy Is Sacred

Keep your energy close to you and protect it. Step away from people and situations that drain you. Let yourself say no when someone asks more of you than you are comfortable giving. Not everyone deserves access to your energy.

☆ .... ☆

DECEMBER 14

Choose Peace

Peace isn't something that just happens. Peace is something you consciously create. Life is a series of choices from the moment you wake up to the moment you fall asleep. Choose peace with every decision you make and watch your world begin to transform.

DECEMBER 15

You Are Sovereign

Do you feel the weight of others' expectations, negativity, and limiting beliefs? You may be highly attuned to the energy of others, but remember that you are a sovereign being. No one can disturb your peace without your permission.

☆ ·· ☆

DECEMBER 16

There Is Beauty in Simplicity

Society wants you to believe that the more you have, the happier you will be. But more is not always better. The less you have, the more time and attention you can dedicate to nurturing what you do have. There is beauty in simplicity.

DECEMBER 17

Invest Wisely

Your time and energy are precious. Be intentional about what you choose to give your attention to and whom you allow access to your energy. Value yourself, create healthy boundaries, and be wise about where you invest your time, energy, and love.

☆ .... ☆

DECEMBER 18

Not Every Feeling Is Yours

Not everything you feel belongs to you. Emotions can be transmitted through family and friends, passed between strangers, even felt from across the globe. Leave your heart open but do not be burdened by that which is not yours to carry.

DECEMBER 19

There Is No Wrong Decision

Life is full of choices, and it can be scary to think that you
took a wrong turn or picked the wrong mountain to climb.
But life is about learning, and there is no such thing as a
wrong decision when your heart is pure.

☆ ·· ☆

DECEMBER 20

Be Mindful

Words carry power. The quality of your thoughts affect
the quality of your life. So, fill your mind, but not with
worry and regret. Fill your mind with words that remind
you of all the wonderful things that you are.

DECEMBER 21

Follow the Magic

Pay attention to what you are drawn to: the magical connection you feel with certain people, places, and things. This feeling is not random. It is here to bring you purpose and peace. Stay close to what makes you feel alive.

☆ ⋯⋯⋯⋯⋯⋯⋯⋯⋯⋯⋯⋯⋯⋯⋯⋯ ☆

DECEMBER 22

Embrace Your Younger Self

Wrap your arms around yourself and envision your younger self. Offer them forgiveness, knowing you did the best you could with the level of awareness you had at the time. And be proud of them, for guiding you toward the compassionate, beautiful, and soulful person you have become.

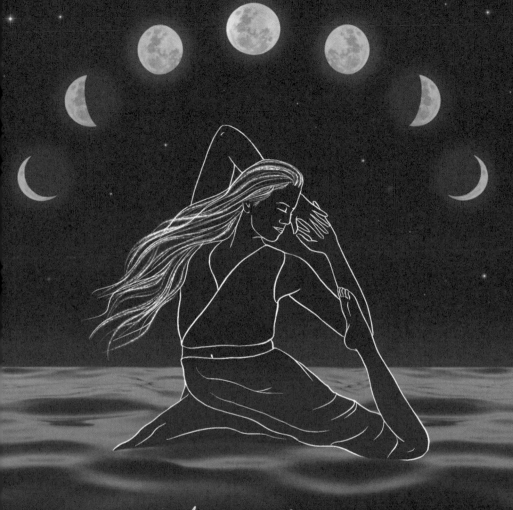

stay close
to what makes you
feel alive

DECEMBER 23
It Can Wait

Whatever thought is playing on repeat in your mind, whatever task you've put on hold, let it be. These things will be okay without you for one night. Take the time you need to rest and restore the health and peace of your mind, body, and spirit.

☆ .... ☆

DECEMBER 24
Seek What You Desire

If you want to feel brave, sit on top of a mountain or swim in the deep ocean. If you want to feel joy, spend time with people who lift your spirits. If you want to feel peace, surround yourself with those who feel like home.

DECEMBER 25

Protect Your Peace

Close your eyes, place your hand on your heart, and say to yourself quietly or out loud, "I am no longer available for situations and people who drain my energy. I respect myself fully. I nurture my mind and body, and I protect my peace."

☆ ·· ☆

DECEMBER 26

Energy Is the Greatest Currency

Everything is energy. And energy is everything. It is the true currency of the Universe and the most valuable thing in this world. Be cautious with things that do not deserve your attention. And be generous with those that do.

DECEMBER 27

Sometimes You Just Know

Sometimes you do not need to be able to explain yourself. There is a voice within you that doesn't speak in words. It speaks in knowingness. It speaks in soul. And that is the only reason you need to listen.

☆ .... ☆

DECEMBER 28

Love Is Freedom

Loving others does not require you to love their beliefs and opinions. You don't have to agree with their choices and actions, either. Let them have their own free will just as you have yours. Love is freedom. This is how the world finds peace.

☆ .... ☆

DECEMBER 29

Remember You Are Peace

There is no doubt the Moon holds a mysterious vibration. Even the most practical person will agree. But the Moon is more than just beautiful to the eye. Next time you gaze up at her, feel her peaceful energy, and remember she reflects you: you are peace, too.

DECEMBER 30

Your Peace Creates Ripples

Your state of being affects so much more than yourself. When you nurture peace within you, you create a domino effect. The peace you've embodied extends outward, finding its way into the hearts of others. And that is how, slowly but surely, the world will find peace.

☆ ⋯⋯⋯⋯⋯⋯⋯⋯⋯⋯⋯⋯⋯⋯⋯ ☆

DECEMBER 31

There Is Magic Here

There is magic to be found here. Pause for a moment and realize how incredible it is that you are awake to your own existence. You are living and breathing and feeling. How miraculous it is simply to be alive.

Acknowledgments

Thank you to my family for always believing in me. Thank you to my friends and Instagram community for their unwavering support and for showing me that soul families exist. And thank you to Rage Kindelsperger, who discovered me, Keyla Pizarro-Hernández, my editor, and everyone else at Quarto who made this book possible.